Mometrix
TEST PREPARATION

Registered Sleep Technologist Exam Secrets Study Guide

Dear Future Exam Success Story

First of all, **THANK YOU** for purchasing Mometrix study materials!

Second, congratulations! You are one of the few determined test-takers who are committed to doing whatever it takes to excel on your exam. **You have come to the right place.** We developed these study materials with one goal in mind: to deliver you the information you need in a format that's concise and easy to use.

In addition to optimizing your guide for the content of the test, we've outlined our recommended steps for breaking down the preparation process into small, attainable goals so you can make sure you stay on track.

We've also analyzed the entire test-taking process, identifying the most common pitfalls and showing how you can overcome them and be ready for any curveball the test throws you.

Standardized testing is one of the biggest obstacles on your road to success, which only increases the importance of doing well in the high-pressure, high-stakes environment of test day. Your results on this test could have a significant impact on your future, and this guide provides the information and practical advice to help you achieve your full potential on test day.

Your success is our success

We would love to hear from you! If you would like to share the story of your exam success or if you have any questions or comments in regard to our products, please contact us at **800-673-8175** or **support@mometrix.com**.

Thanks again for your business and we wish you continued success!

Sincerely,
The Mometrix Test Preparation Team

Written and edited by the Mometrix Exam Secrets Test Prep Team
Printed in the United States of America

TABLE OF CONTENTS

Introduction

Thank you for purchasing this resource! You have made the choice to prepare yourself for a test that could have a huge impact on your future, and this guide is designed to help you be fully ready for test day. Obviously, it's important to have a solid understanding of the test material, but you also need to be prepared for the unique environment and stressors of the test, so that you can perform to the best of your abilities.

For this purpose, the first section that appears in this guide is the **Secret Keys**. We've devoted countless hours to meticulously researching what works and what doesn't, and we've boiled down our findings to the five most impactful steps you can take to improve your performance on the test. We start at the beginning with study planning and move through the preparation process, all the way to the testing strategies that will help you get the most out of what you know when you're finally sitting in front of the test.

We recommend that you start preparing for your test as far in advance as possible. However, if you've bought this guide as a last-minute study resource and only have a few days before your test, we recommend that you skip over the first two Secret Keys since they address a long-term study plan.

If you struggle with **test anxiety**, we strongly encourage you to check out our recommendations for how you can overcome it. Test anxiety is a formidable foe, but it can be beaten, and we want to make sure you have the tools you need to defeat it.

Secret Key #1 – Plan Big, Study Small

There's a lot riding on your performance. If you want to ace this test, you're going to need to keep your skills sharp and the material fresh in your mind. You need a plan that lets you review everything you need to know while still fitting in your schedule. We'll break this strategy down into three categories.

Information Organization

Start with the information you already have: the official test outline. From this, you can make a complete list of all the concepts you need to cover before the test. Organize these concepts into groups that can be studied together, and create a list of any related vocabulary you need to learn so you can brush up on any difficult terms. You'll want to keep this vocabulary list handy once you actually start studying since you may need to add to it along the way.

Time Management

Once you have your set of study concepts, decide how to spread them out over the time you have left before the test. Break your study plan into small, clear goals so you have a manageable task for each day and know exactly what you're doing. Then just focus on one small step at a time. When you manage your time this way, you don't need to spend hours at a time studying. Studying a small block of content for a short period each day helps you retain information better and avoid stressing over how much you have left to do. You can relax knowing that you have a plan to cover everything in time. In order for this strategy to be effective though, you have to start studying early and stick to your schedule. Avoid the exhaustion and futility that comes from last-minute cramming!

Study Environment

The environment you study in has a big impact on your learning. Studying in a coffee shop, while probably more enjoyable, is not likely to be as fruitful as studying in a quiet room. It's important to keep distractions to a minimum. You're only planning to study for a short block of time, so make the most of it. Don't pause to check your phone or get up to find a snack. It's also important to **avoid multitasking**. Research has consistently shown that multitasking will make your studying dramatically less effective. Your study area should also be comfortable and well-lit so you don't have the distraction of straining your eyes or sitting on an uncomfortable chair.

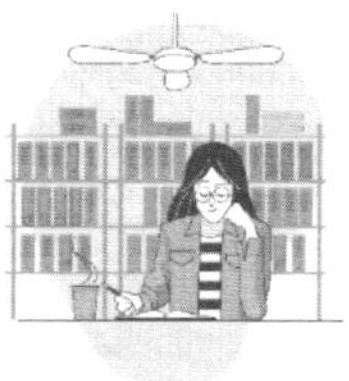

The time of day you study is also important. You want to be rested and alert. Don't wait until just before bedtime. Study when you'll be most likely to comprehend and remember. Even better, if you know what time of day your test will be, set that time aside for study. That way your brain will be used to working on that subject at that specific time and you'll have a better chance of recalling information.

Finally, it can be helpful to team up with others who are studying for the same test. Your actual studying should be done in as isolated an environment as possible, but the work of organizing the information and setting up the study plan can be divided up. In between study sessions, you can discuss with your teammates the concepts that you're all studying and quiz each other on the details. Just be sure that your teammates are as serious about the test as you are. If you find that your study time is being replaced with social time, you might need to find a new team.

Secret Key #2 – Make Your Studying Count

You're devoting a lot of time and effort to preparing for this test, so you want to be absolutely certain it will pay off. This means doing more than just reading the content and hoping you can remember it on test day. It's important to make every minute of study count. There are two main areas you can focus on to make your studying count.

Retention

It doesn't matter how much time you study if you can't remember the material. You need to make sure you are retaining the concepts. To check your retention of the information you're learning, try recalling it at later times with minimal prompting. Try carrying around flashcards and glance at one or two from time to time or ask a friend who's also studying for the test to quiz you.

To enhance your retention, look for ways to put the information into practice so that you can apply it rather than simply recalling it. If you're using the information in practical ways, it will be much easier to remember. Similarly, it helps to solidify a concept in your mind if you're not only reading it to yourself but also explaining it to someone else. Ask a friend to let you teach them about a concept you're a little shaky on (or speak aloud to an imaginary audience if necessary). As you try to summarize, define, give examples, and answer your friend's questions, you'll understand the concepts better and they will stay with you longer. Finally, step back for a big picture view and ask yourself how each piece of information fits with the whole subject. When you link the different concepts together and see them working together as a whole, it's easier to remember the individual components.

Finally, practice showing your work on any multi-step problems, even if you're just studying. Writing out each step you take to solve a problem will help solidify the process in your mind, and you'll be more likely to remember it during the test.

Modality

Modality simply refers to the means or method by which you study. Choosing a study modality that fits your own individual learning style is crucial. No two people learn best in exactly the same way, so it's important to know your strengths and use them to your advantage.

For example, if you learn best by visualization, focus on visualizing a concept in your mind and draw an image or a diagram. Try color-coding your notes, illustrating them, or creating symbols that will trigger your mind to recall a learned concept. If you learn best by hearing or discussing information, find a study partner who learns the same way or read aloud to yourself. Think about how to put the information in your own words. Imagine that you are giving a lecture on the topic and record yourself so you can listen to it later.

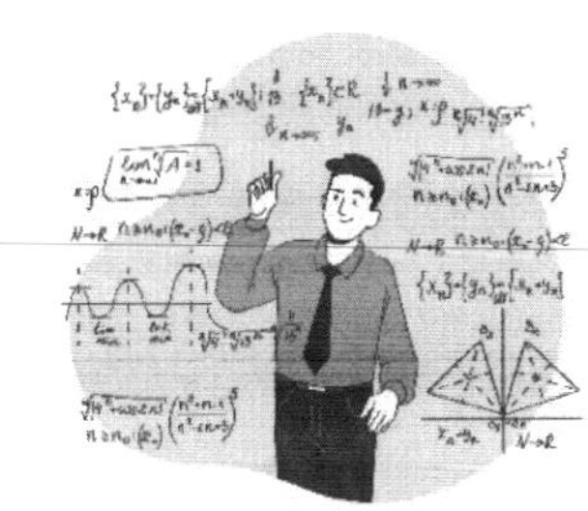

For any learning style, flashcards can be helpful. Organize the information so you can take advantage of spare moments to review. Underline key words or phrases. Use different colors for different categories. Mnemonic devices (such as creating a short list in which every item starts with the same letter) can also help with retention. Find what works best for you and use it to store the information in your mind most effectively and easily.

Secret Key #3 – Practice the Right Way

Your success on test day depends not only on how many hours you put into preparing, but also on whether you prepared the right way. It's good to check along the way to see if your studying is paying off. One of the most effective ways to do this is by taking practice tests to evaluate your progress. Practice tests are useful because they show exactly where you need to improve. Every time you take a practice test, pay special attention to these three groups of questions:

- The questions you got wrong
- The questions you had to guess on, even if you guessed right
- The questions you found difficult or slow to work through

This will show you exactly what your weak areas are, and where you need to devote more study time. Ask yourself why each of these questions gave you trouble. Was it because you didn't understand the material? Was it because you didn't remember the vocabulary? Do you need more repetitions on this type of question to build speed and confidence? Dig into those questions and figure out how you can strengthen your weak areas as you go back to review the material.

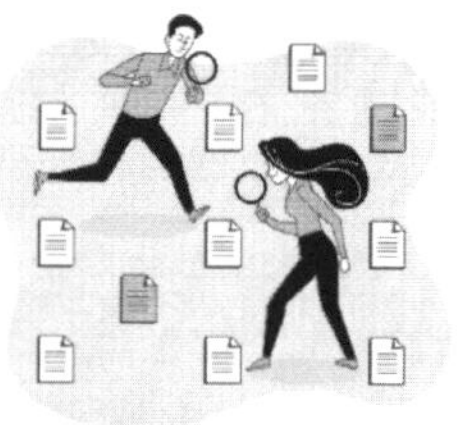

Additionally, many practice tests have a section explaining the answer choices. It can be tempting to read the explanation and think that you now have a good understanding of the concept. However, an explanation likely only covers part of the question's broader context. Even if the explanation makes perfect sense, **go back and investigate** every concept related to the question until you're positive you have a thorough understanding.

As you go along, keep in mind that the practice test is just that: practice. Memorizing these questions and answers will not be very helpful on the actual test because it is unlikely to have any of the same exact questions. If you only know the right answers to the sample questions, you won't be prepared for the real thing. **Study the concepts** until you understand them fully, and then you'll be able to answer any question that shows up on the test.

It's important to wait on the practice tests until you're ready. If you take a test on your first day of study, you may be overwhelmed by the amount of material covered and how much you need to learn. Work up to it gradually.

On test day, you'll need to be prepared for answering questions, managing your time, and using the test-taking strategies you've learned. It's a lot to balance, like a mental marathon that will have a big impact on your future. Like training for a marathon, you'll need to start slowly and work your way up. When test day arrives, you'll be ready.

Start with the strategies you've read in the first two Secret Keys—plan your course and study in the way that works best for you. If you have time, consider using multiple study resources to get different approaches to the same concepts. It can be helpful to see difficult concepts from more than one angle. Then find a good source for practice tests. Many times, the test website will suggest potential study resources or provide sample tests.

Practice Test Strategy

If you're able to find at least three practice tests, we recommend this strategy:

Untimed and Open-Book Practice

Take the first test with no time constraints and with your notes and study guide handy. Take your time and focus on applying the strategies you've learned.

Timed and Open-Book Practice

Take the second practice test open-book as well, but set a timer and practice pacing yourself to finish in time.

Timed and Closed-Book Practice

Take any other practice tests as if it were test day. Set a timer and put away your study materials. Sit at a table or desk in a quiet room, imagine yourself at the testing center, and answer questions as quickly and accurately as possible.

Keep repeating timed and closed-book tests on a regular basis until you run out of practice tests or it's time for the actual test. Your mind will be ready for the schedule and stress of test day, and you'll be able to focus on recalling the material you've learned.

Secret Key #4 – Pace Yourself

Once you're fully prepared for the material on the test, your biggest challenge on test day will be managing your time. Just knowing that the clock is ticking can make you panic even if you have plenty of time left. Work on pacing yourself so you can build confidence against the time constraints of the exam. Pacing is a difficult skill to master, especially in a high-pressure environment, so **practice is vital**.

Set time expectations for your pace based on how much time is available. For example, if a section has 60 questions and the time limit is 30 minutes, you know you have to average 30 seconds or less per question in order to answer them all. Although 30 seconds is the hard limit, set 25 seconds per question as your goal, so you reserve extra time to spend on harder questions. When you budget extra time for the harder questions, you no longer have any reason to stress when those questions take longer to answer.

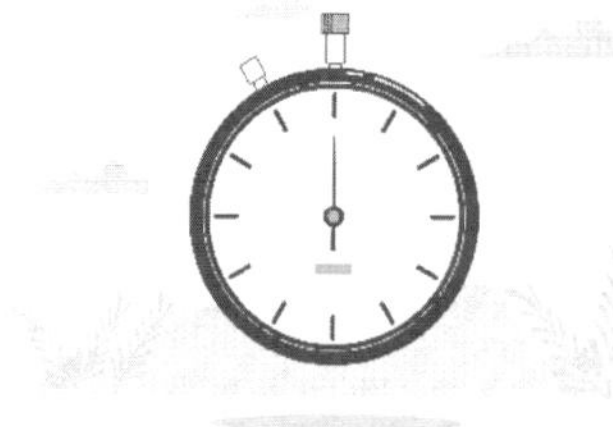

Don't let this time expectation distract you from working through the test at a calm, steady pace, but keep it in mind so you don't spend too much time on any one question. Recognize that taking extra time on one question you don't understand may keep you from answering two that you do understand later in the test. If your time limit for a question is up and you're still not sure of the answer, mark it and move on, and come back to it later if the time and the test format allow. If the testing format doesn't allow you to return to earlier questions, just make an educated guess; then put it out of your mind and move on.

On the easier questions, be careful not to rush. It may seem wise to hurry through them so you have more time for the challenging ones, but it's not worth missing one if you know the concept and just didn't take the time to read the question fully. Work efficiently but make sure you understand the question and have looked at all of the answer choices, since more than one may seem right at first.

Even if you're paying attention to the time, you may find yourself a little behind at some point. You should speed up to get back on track, but do so wisely. Don't panic; just take a few seconds less on each question until you're caught up. Don't guess without thinking, but do look through the answer choices and eliminate any you know are wrong. If you can get down to two choices, it is often worthwhile to guess from those. Once you've chosen an answer, move on and don't dwell on any that you skipped or had to hurry through. If a question was taking too long, chances are it was one of the harder ones, so you weren't as likely to get it right anyway.

On the other hand, if you find yourself getting ahead of schedule, it may be beneficial to slow down a little. The more quickly you work, the more likely you are to make a careless mistake that will affect your score. You've budgeted time for each question, so don't be afraid to spend that time. Practice an efficient but careful pace to get the most out of the time you have.

Secret Key #5 – Have a Plan for Guessing

When you're taking the test, you may find yourself stuck on a question. Some of the answer choices seem better than others, but you don't see the one answer choice that is obviously correct. What do you do?

The scenario described above is very common, yet most test takers have not effectively prepared for it. Developing and practicing a plan for guessing may be one of the single most effective uses of your time as you get ready for the exam.

In developing your plan for guessing, there are three questions to address:

- When should you start the guessing process?
- How should you narrow down the choices?
- Which answer should you choose?

When to Start the Guessing Process

Unless your plan for guessing is to select C every time (which, despite its merits, is not what we recommend), you need to leave yourself enough time to apply your answer elimination strategies. Since you have a limited amount of time for each question, that means that if you're going to give yourself the best shot at guessing correctly, you have to decide quickly whether or not you will guess.

Of course, the best-case scenario is that you don't have to guess at all, so first, see if you can answer the question based on your knowledge of the subject and basic reasoning skills. Focus on the key words in the question and try to jog your memory of related topics. Give yourself a chance to bring the knowledge to mind, but once you realize that you don't have (or you can't access) the knowledge you need to answer the question, it's time to start the guessing process.

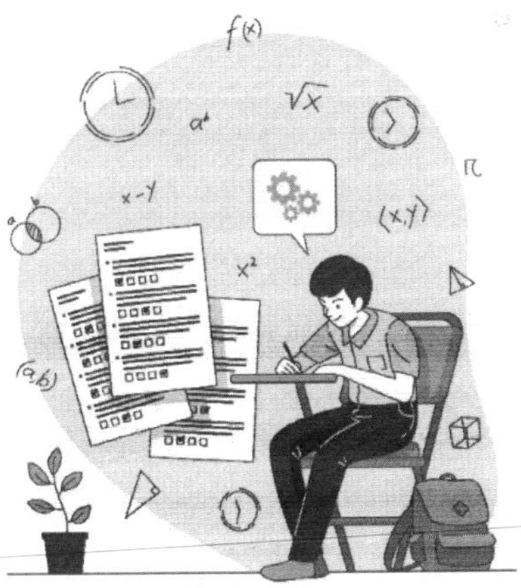

It's almost always better to start the guessing process too early than too late. It only takes a few seconds to remember something and answer the question from knowledge. Carefully eliminating wrong answer choices takes longer. Plus, going through the process of eliminating answer choices can actually help jog your memory.

Summary: Start the guessing process as soon as you decide that you can't answer the question based on your knowledge.

How to Narrow Down the Choices

The next chapter in this book (**Test-Taking Strategies**) includes a wide range of strategies for how to approach questions and how to look for answer choices to eliminate. You will definitely want to read those carefully, practice them, and figure out which ones work best for you. Here though, we're going to address a mindset rather than a particular strategy.

Your odds of guessing an answer correctly depend on how many options you are choosing from.

Number of options left	5	4	3	2	1
Odds of guessing correctly	20%	25%	33%	50%	100%

You can see from this chart just how valuable it is to be able to eliminate incorrect answers and make an educated guess, but there are two things that many test takers do that cause them to miss out on the benefits of guessing:

- Accidentally eliminating the correct answer
- Selecting an answer based on an impression

We'll look at the first one here, and the second one in the next section.

To avoid accidentally eliminating the correct answer, we recommend a thought exercise called **the $5 challenge**. In this challenge, you only eliminate an answer choice from contention if you are willing to bet $5 on it being wrong. Why $5? Five dollars is a small but not insignificant amount of money. It's an amount you could afford to lose but wouldn't want to throw away. And while losing $5 once might not hurt too much, doing it twenty times will set you back $100. In the same way, each small decision you make—eliminating a choice here, guessing on a question there—won't by itself impact your score very much, but when you put them all together, they can make a big difference. By holding each answer choice elimination decision to a higher standard, you can reduce the risk of accidentally eliminating the correct answer.

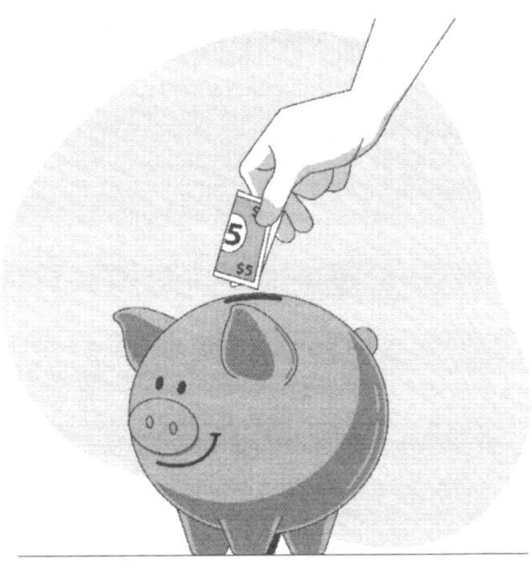

The $5 challenge can also be applied in a positive sense: If you are willing to bet $5 that an answer choice *is* correct, go ahead and mark it as correct.

Summary: Only eliminate an answer choice if you are willing to bet $5 that it is wrong.

Which Answer to Choose

You're taking the test. You've run into a hard question and decided you'll have to guess. You've eliminated all the answer choices you're willing to bet $5 on. Now you have to pick an answer. Why do we even need to talk about this? Why can't you just pick whichever one you feel like when the time comes?

The answer to these questions is that if you don't come into the test with a plan, you'll rely on your impression to select an answer choice, and if you do that, you risk falling into a trap. The test writers know that everyone who takes their test will be guessing on some of the questions, so they intentionally write wrong answer choices to seem plausible. You still have to pick an answer though, and if the wrong answer choices are designed to look right, how can you ever be sure that you're not falling for their trap? The best solution we've found to this dilemma is to take the decision out of your hands entirely. Here is the process we recommend:

Once you've eliminated any choices that you are confident (willing to bet $5) are wrong, select the first remaining choice as your answer.

Whether you choose to select the first remaining choice, the second, or the last, the important thing is that you use some preselected standard. Using this approach guarantees that you will not be enticed into selecting an answer choice that looks right, because you are not basing your decision on how the answer choices look.

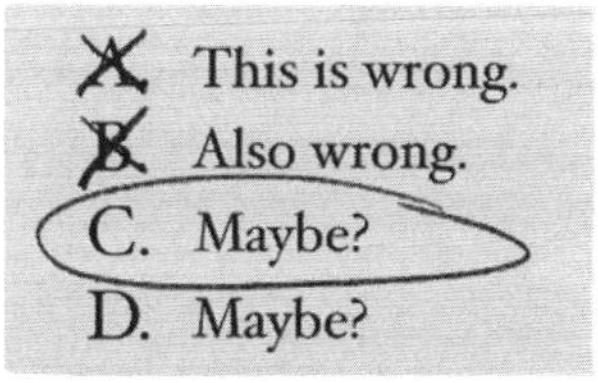

This is not meant to make you question your knowledge. Instead, it is to help you recognize the difference between your knowledge and your impressions. There's a huge difference between thinking an answer is right because of what you know, and thinking an answer is right because it looks or sounds like it should be right.

Summary: To ensure that your selection is appropriately random, make a predetermined selection from among all answer choices you have not eliminated.

Test-Taking Strategies

This section contains a list of test-taking strategies that you may find helpful as you work through the test. By taking what you know and applying logical thought, you can maximize your chances of answering any question correctly!

It is very important to realize that every question is different and every person is different: no single strategy will work on every question, and no single strategy will work for every person. That's why we've included all of them here, so you can try them out and determine which ones work best for different types of questions and which ones work best for you.

Question Strategies

☑ Read Carefully

Read the question and the answer choices carefully. Don't miss the question because you misread the terms. You have plenty of time to read each question thoroughly and make sure you understand what is being asked. Yet a happy medium must be attained, so don't waste too much time. You must read carefully and efficiently.

☑ Contextual Clues

Look for contextual clues. If the question includes a word you are not familiar with, look at the immediate context for some indication of what the word might mean. Contextual clues can often give you all the information you need to decipher the meaning of an unfamiliar word. Even if you can't determine the meaning, you may be able to narrow down the possibilities enough to make a solid guess at the answer to the question.

☑ Prefixes

If you're having trouble with a word in the question or answer choices, try dissecting it. Take advantage of every clue that the word might include. Prefixes can be a huge help. Usually, they allow you to determine a basic meaning. *Pre-* means before, *post-* means after, *pro-* is positive, *de-* is negative. From prefixes, you can get an idea of the general meaning of the word and try to put it into context.

☑ Hedge Words

Watch out for critical hedge words, such as *likely, may, can, often, almost, mostly, usually, generally, rarely,* and *sometimes.* Question writers insert these hedge phrases to cover every possibility. Often an answer choice will be wrong simply because it leaves no room for exception. Be on guard for answer choices that have definitive words such as *exactly* and *always.*

☑ Switchback Words

Stay alert for *switchbacks.* These are the words and phrases frequently used to alert you to shifts in thought. The most common switchback words are *but, although,* and *however.* Others include *nevertheless, on the other hand, even though, while, in spite of, despite,* and *regardless of.* Switchback words are important to catch because they can change the direction of the question or an answer choice.

✅ Face Value

When in doubt, use common sense. Accept the situation in the problem at face value. Don't read too much into it. These problems will not require you to make wild assumptions. If you have to go beyond creativity and warp time or space in order to have an answer choice fit the question, then you should move on and consider the other answer choices. These are normal problems rooted in reality. The applicable relationship or explanation may not be readily apparent, but it is there for you to figure out. Use your common sense to interpret anything that isn't clear.

Answer Choice Strategies

✅ Answer Selection

The most thorough way to pick an answer choice is to identify and eliminate wrong answers until only one is left, then confirm it is the correct answer. Sometimes an answer choice may immediately seem right, but be careful. The test writers will usually put more than one reasonable answer choice on each question, so take a second to read all of them and make sure that the other choices are not equally obvious. As long as you have time left, it is better to read every answer choice than to pick the first one that looks right without checking the others.

✅ Answer Choice Families

An answer choice family consists of two (in rare cases, three) answer choices that are very similar in construction and cannot all be true at the same time. If you see two answer choices that are direct opposites or parallels, one of them is usually the correct answer. For instance, if one answer choice says that quantity *x* increases and another either says that quantity *x* decreases (opposite) or says that quantity *y* increases (parallel), then those answer choices would fall into the same family. An answer choice that doesn't match the construction of the answer choice family is more likely to be incorrect. Most questions will not have answer choice families, but when they do appear, you should be prepared to recognize them.

✅ Eliminate Answers

Eliminate answer choices as soon as you realize they are wrong, but make sure you consider all possibilities. If you are eliminating answer choices and realize that the last one you are left with is also wrong, don't panic. Start over and consider each choice again. There may be something you missed the first time that you will realize on the second pass.

✅ Avoid Fact Traps

Don't be distracted by an answer choice that is factually true but doesn't answer the question. You are looking for the choice that answers the question. Stay focused on what the question is asking for so you don't accidentally pick an answer that is true but incorrect. Always go back to the question and make sure the answer choice you've selected actually answers the question and is not merely a true statement.

✅ Extreme Statements

In general, you should avoid answers that put forth extreme actions as standard practice or proclaim controversial ideas as established fact. An answer choice that states the "process should be used in certain situations, if..." is much more likely to be correct than one that states the "process should be discontinued completely." The first is a calm rational statement and doesn't even make a definitive, uncompromising stance, using a hedge word *if* to provide wiggle room, whereas the second choice is far more extreme.

⊘ Benchmark

As you read through the answer choices and you come across one that seems to answer the question well, mentally select that answer choice. This is not your final answer, but it's the one that will help you evaluate the other answer choices. The one that you selected is your benchmark or standard for judging each of the other answer choices. Every other answer choice must be compared to your benchmark. That choice is correct until proven otherwise by another answer choice beating it. If you find a better answer, then that one becomes your new benchmark. Once you've decided that no other choice answers the question as well as your benchmark, you have your final answer.

⊘ Predict the Answer

Before you even start looking at the answer choices, it is often best to try to predict the answer. When you come up with the answer on your own, it is easier to avoid distractions and traps because you will know exactly what to look for. The right answer choice is unlikely to be word-for-word what you came up with, but it should be a close match. Even if you are confident that you have the right answer, you should still take the time to read each option before moving on.

General Strategies

⊘ Tough Questions

If you are stumped on a problem or it appears too hard or too difficult, don't waste time. Move on! Remember though, if you can quickly check for obviously incorrect answer choices, your chances of guessing correctly are greatly improved. Before you completely give up, at least try to knock out a couple of possible answers. Eliminate what you can and then guess at the remaining answer choices before moving on.

⊘ Check Your Work

Since you will probably not know every term listed and the answer to every question, it is important that you get credit for the ones that you do know. Don't miss any questions through careless mistakes. If at all possible, try to take a second to look back over your answer selection and make sure you've selected the correct answer choice and haven't made a costly careless mistake (such as marking an answer choice that you didn't mean to mark). This quick double check should more than pay for itself in caught mistakes for the time it costs.

⊘ Pace Yourself

It's easy to be overwhelmed when you're looking at a page full of questions; your mind is confused and full of random thoughts, and the clock is ticking down faster than you would like. Calm down and maintain the pace that you have set for yourself. Especially as you get down to the last few minutes of the test, don't let the small numbers on the clock make you panic. As long as you are on track by monitoring your pace, you are guaranteed to have time for each question.

⊘ Don't Rush

It is very easy to make errors when you are in a hurry. Maintaining a fast pace in answering questions is pointless if it makes you miss questions that you would have gotten right otherwise. Test writers like to include distracting information and wrong answers that seem right. Taking a little extra time to avoid careless mistakes can make all the difference in your test score. Find a pace that allows you to be confident in the answers that you select.

✓ KEEP MOVING

Panicking will not help you pass the test, so do your best to stay calm and keep moving. Taking deep breaths and going through the answer elimination steps you practiced can help to break through a stress barrier and keep your pace.

Final Notes

The combination of a solid foundation of content knowledge and the confidence that comes from practicing your plan for applying that knowledge is the key to maximizing your performance on test day. As your foundation of content knowledge is built up and strengthened, you'll find that the strategies included in this chapter become more and more effective in helping you quickly sift through the distractions and traps of the test to isolate the correct answer.

Now that you're preparing to move forward into the test content chapters of this book, be sure to keep your goal in mind. As you read, think about how you will be able to apply this information on the test. If you've already seen sample questions for the test and you have an idea of the question format and style, try to come up with questions of your own that you can answer based on what you're reading. This will give you valuable practice applying your knowledge in the same ways you can expect to on test day.

Good luck and good studying!

Study Performance

Selecting Equipment and Montage

Patient Rooms

Patient rooms vary considerably but should be as non-institution-like as possible with at least 140 square feet recommended for each patient. The bed should be positioned so that staff can access the patient on both sides. Adjustable beds provide more comfort to help patients relax. Blackout blinds should be available to block outside lights at night and ambient daylight for daytime napping. When possible, the day and nighttime room temperatures should be set to the patient's preference. Fans or extra blankets should be available if individual room temperatures cannot be set. Restrooms should be clean and easily available to the patient. Shared bathrooms must be monitored and cleaned frequently. Storage space should be adequate to contain patient's clothing and toiletries as well as equipment and supplies needed during testing. If showers are available for patient use, they should be stocked with individual soap, shampoo, and towels.

Electroencephalogram

Electroencephalograms (EEGs) measure the electrical activity within the brain through scalp electrodes to rule out seizure disorders and to determine the characteristics of the sleep-wake state. Waves/cycles in 1 second are measured in Hertz (Hz) to determine the stage of sleep:

- Alpha: 8–13 Hz
- Beta: 13–30 Hz
- Delta: < 0.5–4 Hz
- Theta: > 4–7 Hz

The EEG equipment may be analog, with waves recorded on paper, or digital, with waves recorded electronically for viewing on a computer screen. All equipment should be properly calibrated, and paper should be inserted before use (for analog). Digital EEG equipment is usually used instead of analog because it presents a more accurate reading and allows a variety of filters for different montages. The EEG can be set to display the electroencephalograph in page mode (usually showing 10-second increments) or in continuous scroll mode. Typically, six leads are used (including two reference leads) although more may be applied to diagnose seizure disorders.

Face Electrodes

Face electrodes are used to ground and to record eye and chin activity and include:

- Ground electrode: This electrode does not impact measurements with modern computerized equipment. It is usually placed in the middle of the forehead but can be placed anywhere on the body.
- Electrooculogram (EOG): The EOG records vertical and horizontal eye movements and helps to identify periods of REM sleep. A pair of electrodes is placed with one electrode by the right eye and the other by the left.
- Chin electromyogram (cEMG): The cEMG records muscle tone of the chin muscles and helps to identify REM sleep, during which muscle tone decreases. The cEMG can also provide information about teeth grinding, which causes muscle movement, and snoring, as snoring causes artifacts.

Electrocardiogram

Electrocardiograms (ECGs) record and show a graphic display of the electrical activity of the heart through a number of different waveforms, complexes, and intervals:

- P wave: The P wave represents the beginning of electrical impulses in the sinus node, which spread through the atria (muscle depolarization).
- QRS complex: The QRS complex represents ventricular muscle depolarization and atrial repolarization.
- T wave: The T wave represents ventricular muscle repolarization (resting state) as cells regain negative charge.
- U wave: The U wave represents repolarization of the Purkinje fibers.

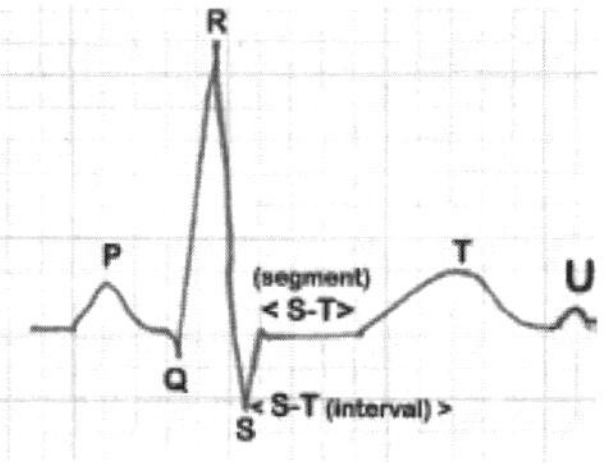

A modified lead II ECG is typically used for polysomnography to identify basic heart rhythms and dysrhythmias. Typical placement of leads for a 2-lead ECG is 3–5 cm inferior to the right clavicle and left lower ribcage. Typical placement for a 3-lead ECG is the right arm near the shoulder (RA), V_5 position over the 5th intercostal space (LA), and the left upper leg near the groin (LL).

Anterior Tibialis Electromyogram

Anterior tibialis electromyograms (atEMGs) monitor the electrical activity in the leg muscles, allowing for monitoring of periodic leg movement during the polysomnogram because electrical activity is absent when the muscle is relaxed and increases with movement. The atEMG may show twitching and slight muscle activity and movement that may not be obvious by observation alone. Typically, muscle activity slows during sleep, especially during REM sleep so that people are not active while dreaming. While intramuscular leads are used to diagnose neuromuscular disorders, surface leads are used for polysomnography because only a general overview of muscle activity is needed. In some cases, if respiratory effort is being monitored, leads may be placed intercostally.

Sensors

Sensors may be used during the polysomnogram to provide additional information about breathing during sleep:

- Respiratory effort: Piezo-sensor bands or respiratory inductive plethysmography are used to indicate chest and abdominal movement during respiration as an indirect means of representing respiratory effort.
- Snore: Microphones or piezo-sensors applied to the lateral-anterior neck superior to the larynx are used to indicate the degree and duration of snoring. Sensors are more accurate than microphones.
- Airflow: Thermal sensors (thermistors or thermocouples) or pressure transducers (nasal) monitor both intake and outflow of air through the nostrils and the mouth. Typically, two prongs are inserted into the nose and a third prong is in front of the mouth.

Pulse Oximetry

Pulse oximetry, continuous or intermittent, uses an external oximeter that attaches to the patient's finger (or earlobe) to measure arterial oxygen saturation (SpO_2), the percentage of hemoglobin that is saturated with oxygen. The oximeter also indicates the current heart rate. The oximeter uses light waves to determine SpO_2. Normal SpO_2 should be over 95% although some patients with chronic respiratory disorders, such as chronic obstructive pulmonary disease may have lower SpO_2 values. Impaired circulation, excessive light, poor positioning, and nail polish may compromise results. If SpO_2 falls, the oximeter should be repositioned, as an incorrect position is a common cause of inaccurate readings. Oximeters do not provide information about carbon dioxide levels, so they cannot monitor carbon dioxide retention. The oximeter is usually placed on an index finger but may be placed on an earlobe if necessary.

Inspection of Equipment

Inspection of equipment should precede the examination. Before beginning the polysomnogram, the equipment is thoroughly inspected to ensure that the system is connected to electricity, that all cables and wires are secure, and that the equipment is functioning properly. The computer is turned on, and the patient information file is opened to ensure that information about the patient was entered correctly into the system. Any equipment issues, such as malfunctioning or incompatibility, are resolved before beginning the test as this may impact the results. All necessary supplies and equipment, such as leads, glue, and tape, are laid out and easily accessible to avoid unnecessary delays, thereby reducing patient stress. The physician's orders should be checked to verify that the correct montage has been selected.

Selection of Montage

Selection of the montage depends on the presumptive diagnosis and the type of testing.

Nocturnal polysomnogram (PSG)	EEG, EOG, cEMG, atEMG, pulse oximetry, and sensors for respiratory effort, snore, and airflow.	Used to diagnose obstructive sleep apnea syndrome and may be done before MSLT.
Multiple sleep latency test (MSLT)	EEG (central and occipital), EOG cEMG, and ECG; other channels are optional.	Used to diagnose excessive sleepiness (hypersomnia) and narcolepsy during waking hours; done after nocturnal PSG to ensure 6 hours of sleep preceding test.
Maintenance of wakeful-ness test	Same as for MSLT.	Used to evaluate success of treatment or ability to stay awake during the daytime; does not usually require a nocturnal PSG although it may be indicated for shift workers.

Abbreviations: EEG = electroencephalogram; EOG = electrooculogram; cEMG = chin electromyogram; atEMG = anterior tibialis electromyogram; and ECG = electrocardiogram

Applying Sensors

Electroencephalogram Electrodes and Sensors

Electroencephalogram (EEG) electrodes and sensors must be applied properly in the correct position. EEG electrodes are placed using the international 10/20 measuring system, which uses the nasion, inion, and preauricular points as landmarks while measuring the skull to determine lead placement at 10%–20% distance from the landmarks. EEG leads are designated, according to the part of the skull to which they are applied, with even numbered subscripts on the right and odd numbered subscripts on the left. The system reference electrode is placed according to software requirements, often the central lead (C_z) at the vertex or top center of the head. Sleep technology often requires only a modified EEG with fewer electrodes, typically right and left central (C_4 and C_3), right and left occipital (O_2 and O_1), and right and left reference mastoid leads (A_2 and A_1).

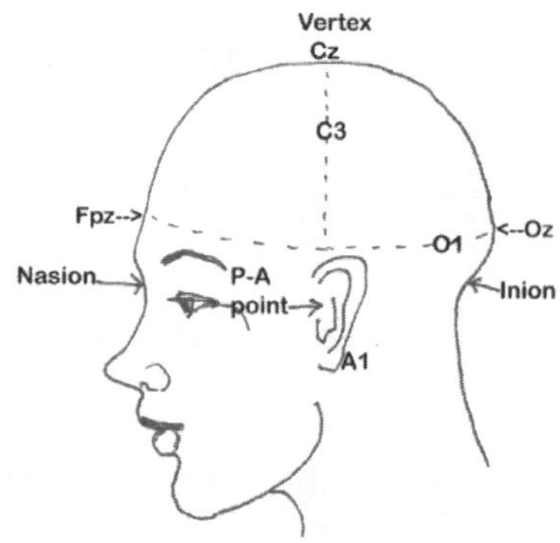

Scalp Electrode Site Measuring

Scalp electrode site measuring uses the international 10/20 measuring system based on landmarks (e.g., nasion, inion, preauricular points). Sleep technicians must be proficient at performing these site measurements. Points are labeled, according to area of the brain and the exact site, so O_1 is occipital area 1 with odd numbers indicating the left side:

C_z is measured vertically from the inion to the nasion and midline. The technician marks the 50% (vertex) measure at the top of the head as well as a 10% and two 20% measures on each side of the vertex, starting at the nasion and inion. The technician then measures from the left preauricular point to the right, intersecting at the 50% mark (vertex) and marking a 10% and two 20% measures on each side of the vertex, starting at the preauricular points. The point where the two vertical lines intersect at the vertex is C_z.

Other scalp electrode sites are measured once the vertical lines connecting the nasion and inion and the preauricular points are drawn and C_z is identified. The technologist measures the following:

- Fpz and Oz: A vertical line is drawn 10% superior to the nasion, midline, to identify Fpz and 10% superior to the inion to identify Oz. A horizontal line is drawn 10% above the preauricular points to create a horizontal line that circles the head through Oz and Fpz.
- C3: On the 30% mark (10% plus 20%) above the left preauricular point
- C4: On the 30% mark (10% plus 20%) above the right preauricular point
- O1: On the 5% mark to the left of Oz on the horizontal line that is 10% above the left preauricular point
- O2: On the 5% mark to the right of Oz on the horizontal line that is10% above the right preauricular point
- A1: Over the left mastoid process behind ear
- A2: Over the right mastoid process behind ear

Face, Electrooculogram, and Chin Electromyogram Electrode Placement

Face, electrooculogram (EOG), and chin electromyogram (cEMG) electrode placement during polysomnography include the following:

Ground electrode	Place electrode on central forehead on line between nasion and hairline on a flat area of skin, avoiding deep wrinkles or creases.
EOG	Right electrode: Place electrode 1 cm lateral to and 1 cm superior to the outer canthus.
	Left electrode: Place electrode 1 cm lateral to and 1 cm inferior to the outer canthus.
cEMG	Method 1: Place two electrodes on chin, 3 cm apart and 2 cm below lower lip.
	Method 2: Place two electrodes on submentalis muscle, 3 cm apart (advised for thin but not obese patients).
	Method 3: Place one electrode on the chin (center) and the other on the submentalis muscle.
Anterior tibialis electromyogram	Place two electrodes 3 cm apart along the anterior tibialis ridges on both legs, avoiding the tibias.

Respiratory Effort, Snore, Airflow, and Oximeter

Sensors, such as respiratory effort, snore, airflow, and oximeter, are used during polysomnography.

Respiratory effort	Bands (sized for the individual patient) containing sensors are placed securely (being careful not to restrict breathing) about the patient's body with lead wires pointed upwards: Thorax: Secured just below axilla Abdomen: Secured about the waist
Snore	Microphone: Placed close to the patient
	Sensor: Placed laterally on the anterior neck, superior to the larynx
Airflow	Nasal prongs are inserted into the nostrils, and the third prong is positioned in front of the mouth.
Oximeter	The oximeter is clipped to the index finger closest to oximeter or to the earlobe.

Head and Face Electrode Sites

Head and face electrodes are applied to areas that are clean and free of oil to ensure good quality signals. Before attachment, the skin must be cleaned thoroughly with an alcohol swab and then scrubbed for 5–10 seconds with an abrasive skin cleanser, such as NuPrep, using a cotton swab and being sure to scrub only the area of attachment, carefully separating the hair on the scalp.

Collodion Attachment

Collodion attachment involves placing the electrode on the scrubbed site and covered with 2–3-cm size square of single-ply gauze. The air compressor stylus is inserted through the gauze and into the top center of the electrode and then collodion glue is applied with an eyedropper to saturate the gauze. Smooth gauze is placed over the scalp or skin while drying with an air compressor, using care to avoid getting glue between the electrode and the skin. The stylus is removed. Using a blunt-tipped needle, the electrode is filled with electrolyte gel/cream.

Electrode Cream and Tape Attachment

Head and face electrodes are applied by different methods after the skin is scrubbed, including:

- Electrode cream attachment: Electrode cream (EC2), which is an adhesive, is applied to one side of a 3-cm square of single-ply gauze. The electrode cup is filled with electrolyte paste/conductive gel, and the lead is placed in the middle of the gauze (gel side facing upward) to secure it to the gauze; the electrode and the gauze are then inverted onto the scrubbed skin, smoothing the gauze over the skin to secure it.
- Electrode tape attachment (electrode collar): The electrode cup is filled with electrolyte paste/conductive gel and inverted onto the skin. The electrode is covered with tape, which is smoothed to secure it to the skin. The electrode is tucked under a corner of the tape to facilitate later removal.

Electrode leads from the face and scalp should be gathered together and secured with tape or Velcro every 4–6 inches to prevent tangling.

Body Electrode Sites

Body electrode sites include those for the electrocardiogram (ECG) and the anterior tibialis electromyogram (atEMG). Applying the electrodes includes:

- Skin preparation: Electrode placement sites are thoroughly cleaned with alcohol, using a cotton applicator or premoistened alcohol swab. An abrasive cleaner, such as NuPrep, is indicated only if impedance is high. If the patient is hairy (primarily men), the area may need to be shaved before cleaning the skin.
- Application:
    - ECG: The lead wire is attached to the electrode before application. The adhesive backing is removed, and the gel side is placed against the skin, feeding the wires through the patient's clothing, and then plugging them into the appropriate jack.
    - atEMG: Electrodes are attached with a double-sided electrode collar and taped (2 inches). The electrode wires are looped between the electrodes and secured to prevent dislodgment during the exam.

Verifying Impedances

Verifying impedances is done by the technologist after calibrating the machine to determine if the electrodes are properly applied and signal quality is appropriate. Electrodes pick up the electrical current generated by tissue and transmit this signal to the machine, which creates a wave pattern. If the connection between the electrode and the conducting gel is disrupted, the signal is distorted, causing motion artifacts. Silver/silver chloride electrodes tend to have less motion artifacts than gold electrodes. Impedance refers to interference with the electrical signal from the point of contact to the recording device. Each type of electrode has an associated source impedance, but impedance levels for each individual electrode should remain low ($\leq$ 5 kilohms). Each electrode should be individually tested, using the internal impedance meter or an external handheld meter. A difference in impedance between paired electrodes increases artifacts. If the impedance level of an electrode is high, then the electrode may need to be repositioned.

Educating Patients

Patient Orientation

Patient orientation begins with the patient's arrival at the facility. Orientation should include:

- Introduction: The patient should be introduced to the technologist and any other staff members who may be present. This is especially important if the patient is to be awakened.
- Tour of physical plant: The initial tour should include the patient's individual sleeping area and storage space as well as the bathroom and shower facilities. The patient should observe the technologist's monitoring area and any monitoring equipment.
- Equipment: The technologist should identify and explain the bedside equipment used to monitor sleep.
- Alarms: Any alarms or call bells should be demonstrated so the patient knows how to use them and recognizes the sound.
- Lights/fans: The patient should know the location of light switches, temperature controls (if available), and fans and should receive instructions on their use.
- Patient's rights: The technologist should apprise the patient of his or her rights, including the right to privacy and confidentiality and the right to refuse treatment, according to the rules of the Health Insurance Portability and Accountability Act.

Learning Styles

Learning styles—visual, auditory, and kinesthetic—differ among patients, and not all people are aware of their preferences. A range of teaching materials/methods that relates to all three learning preferences and are age-appropriate should be available. Part of assessment for teaching involves choosing the right approach based on observation and feedback. Often presenting learners with different options gives a clue to their preferred learning style. Some people have a combined learning style.

Visual learners	Learn best by seeing and reading: Provide written directions or picture guides and demonstrate procedures. Use charts and diagrams. Provide photos and videos.
Auditory learners	Learn best by listening and talking:Procedures while demonstrating and have learner repeat. Plan extra time to discuss and answer questions. Provide audiotapes.
Kinesthetic learners	Learn best by handling, doing, and practicing: Provide hands-on experience throughout teaching. Encourage handling of supplies/equipment. Allow learner to demonstrate. Minimize instructions and allow person to explore equipment and procedures.

Handouts

Handouts are commonly used to teach patients; to be sure that they do not end up in the wastebasket without ever being read, these handouts should follow the following pointers:

- Handouts that simply copy a slide show presentation or repeat everything in the presentation are less helpful than those that summarize the main points.
- Providing handouts immediately before a discussion often results in the patient looking at the handout instead of the speaker. Thus, handouts should either be given to the patient before instruction so they can be reviewed in advance or passed out at the end of the meeting.
- Poster-type handouts (with drawings or pictures) that can be placed on bulletin boards are useful.
- Handouts should be easily readable and not smudged copies of newspaper articles or small print text.

Videos

Videos are a useful adjunct to teaching as they reduce the time needed for one-on-one instruction (increasing cost-effectiveness). Passive presentation of videos, such as in the waiting area, has little value, but focused viewing in which the technologist discusses the purpose of the video presentation before viewing and then is available for discussion after viewing can be very effective. Patients or families are often nervous about testing and are unsure of their role, so they may not focus completely when the technologist is presenting information. Allowing the patients and families to watch a video demonstration or explanation first and allowing them to stop or review the video presentation can help them to grasp the fundamentals before they have to apply them, relieving some of the anxiety they may be experiencing. Videos are much more effective than written materials for those with low literacy or poor English skills. The technologist should always be available to answer questions and discuss the material after the patients and families finish viewing.

Readability

Readability (the grade level of material) is a concern because many patients and families may have limited English skills or low literacy, and it can be difficult for the technologist to assess people's reading level. Studies have indicated that learning is more effective if oral presentations and demonstrations are supplemented with reading materials, such as handouts. The average American reads effectively at the 6th to 8th grade level (regardless of education achieved), but many health education materials have a much higher readability level. Additionally, research indicates that even people with much higher reading skills learn medical and health information most effectively when the material is presented at the 6th to 8th grade readability level. Therefore, patient education materials (and consent forms) should not be written at higher than 6th to 8th grade level. Readability index calculators are available on the Internet to give an approximation of grade level and difficulty for those preparing materials without expertise in reading.

Bloom's Taxonomy and Three Types of Learning

Bloom's taxonomy outlines behaviors that are necessary for learning and describes three types of learning: cognitive, affective, and psychomotor.

Cognitive	Knowledge
	Comprehension
	Application
	Analysis

(learning and gaining intellectual skills to master six categories of effective learning)	Synthesis
	Evaluation
Affective (recognizing five categories of feelings and values from simple to complex; slower to achieve than cognitive learning)	Receiving phenomena: Accepts the need to learn
	Responding to phenomena: Takes an active part in care
	Valuing: Understands value of becoming independent in care
	Organizing values: Understands how surgery or treatment has improved life
	Internalizing values: Accepts condition as part of life; is consistent and self-reliant
Psychomotor(mastering six motor skills necessary for independence; follows a progression from simple to complex)	Perception: Uses sensory information to learn tasks
	Set: Shows willingness to perform tasks
	Guided response: Follows directions
	Mechanism: Does specific tasks
	Complex overt response: Displays competence in self-care
	Adaptation: Modifies procedures as needed
	Origination: Creatively deals with problems

Knowles' Theory of Andragogy

Knowles' theory of andragogy pertains to adult learners who are more interested in process than in information and content. Knowles outlined some principles of adult learning and typical characteristics of adult learners.

Practical and goal-oriented	Provide overviews or summaries and examples.
	Use collaborative discussions with problem-solving exercises.
	Remain organized with the goal in mind.
Self-directed	Provide active involvement, asking for input.
	Allow different options toward achieving the goal.
	Give them responsibilities.
Knowledgeable	Show respect for their life experiences and education.
	Validate their knowledge, and ask for feedback.New material to information with which they are familiar.
Relevancy-oriented	Explain how information will be applied.
	Clearly identify objectives.
Motivated	Provide certificates of achievement or some type of recognition for achievement.

Teaching Older Adults

Teaching older adults can be accomplished with a number of strategies.

- Spend a little time getting to know the patient so that he or she is more relaxed and receptive to learning.
- Determine what information is critical for the patient to learn and what is nonessential.
- Evaluate the patient's learning style and previous knowledge about the topic.
- Plan for ample time for each session of instruction, and plan the probable number of sessions to determine how much instruction will be needed for each session. Ensure that sessions are closely spaced to reinforce learning.
- Provide the patient ample time to practice.
- Allow the patient to guide the pace of the session as much as possible, and encourage feedback.
- Prepare age-appropriate handouts at an accessible reading level and with large-size font.
- Provide materials (e.g., pencil, paper) in case the patient wants to make notes.
- Be supportive, patient, and enthusiastic.

Readiness to Learn: Physical Factors and Experience

Readiness to learn on the part of the patient and family is assessed because if a person is not ready, instruction is of little value. Often readiness is indicated when the patient and family ask questions or show an interest in procedures. There are a number of factors related to readiness to learn.

- Physical factors: There are a number of physical factors than can affect ability. Manual dexterity may be required to complete a task, and this varies with age and physical condition. Hearing or vision deficits may impact ability. Complex tasks may be too difficult for some because of weakness or cognitive impairment, and modifications of the environment may be needed. Health status, age, and gender may all impact the ability to learn.
- Experience: People's experience with learning varies widely and is affected by their ability to cope with changes, their personal goals, motivation to learn, and cultural background. People may have widely divergent ideas about what constitutes illness or treatment. Lack of English skills may make learning difficult and prevent people from asking questions.

Readiness to learn includes:

- Mental/emotional status: The support system and motivation may impact readiness. Anxiety, fear, or depression about a physical condition can make learning very difficult because the patient or family cannot focus on learning; thus, the technologist must spend time to reassure the patient and family and wait until they are emotionally more receptive.
- Knowledge/education: The knowledge base of the patient and family, their cognitive ability, and their learning styles all affect their readiness to learn. The technologist begins by assessing what knowledge the patient and family already have about the disease, condition, or treatment and then builds from that base. People with little medical experience may lack knowledge of basic medical terminology, which may interfere with their ability and readiness to learn.

Physical Disabilities

Cognitive Impairment

Cognitive impairment can be challenging, and patients may have very individual responses, so observation of the patient must serve as a guide. Patients may be apprehensive and frightened, so the technologist maintains a friendly normal tone of voice and speaks with the patient often to establish rapport, even if the response is not clear. The technologist always asks the patient before touching his or her things. Initiating communication by talking about familiar things (e.g., family, pictures, the past) may be comforting for the patient. If responses are unclear or inappropriate, the technologist can say, "I didn't understand that" but should not laugh or indicate frustration. The technologist should face the patient and maintain eye contact to help the patient stay focused. Patients may get up and move away or go for a walk, and the technologist should not try to restrain the patient but should ask if he or she can walk with the person.

Hearing-Impaired and Deaf Patients

Hearing-impaired patients may have some hearing and may use hearing aids, while deaf patients typically have little or no hearing. Some patients are able to lip-read to various degrees; thus, the technologist should always face the patient within 3–6 feet and speak slowly and clearly, using gestures (not excessively) to augment speech:

- Hearing impaired: Assistive devices (e.g., hearing aids, writing material) should be available and used during communication. A normal tone of voice and short sentences are effective. Environmental noises are minimized.
- Deaf: If patients are deaf, sign language interpreters are used for important communications; the interviewer should face the patient, not the interpreter. Assistive devices, such as writing materials, TDD phone/relay service, should also be available for use. The technologist should always announce his or her presence on entering a room by waving, clapping, or tapping the foot (whatever works best for the patient). It is important to ensure alarms have visual feedback (lights), and technologists should not chew, smoke, or eat while speaking to the patient.

Visual Impairment

Visual impairment is unrelated to intelligence or hearing, so the technologist should speak with age-appropriate vocabulary in a normal tone of voice, facing the patient so the technologist can observe facial expressions. Depending on the degree of visual impairment, the patient may not be able to see gestures or materials; so alternate forms of materials (braille handouts or enlarged text) or manipulatives must be considered. The field of vision may be impaired so that the patient sees shapes or has better vision in some areas than others; thus, the technologist should try to position him- or herself for the patient's advantage. The technologist should also announce his or her presence, explain actions and movement ("I am putting your supplies in the drawer"), announce position ("I am at your right side") and always tell the patient if the technologist is going to touch the patient ("I am going to apply an electrode to your right leg").

Equipment Calibration

Equipment Calibration Before and After Exam

Equipment calibration (with standard settings for filters and sensitivity) of 30 seconds must be done and recorded before beginning the polysomnogram after the leads and sensors are applied and the patient is quiet. Calibration procedures vary somewhat, depending on the software and equipment used, so manufacturer's instructions should be noted and followed. Electroencephalograms, electrooculograms, and electromyograms generally require negative 50 microvolts per centimeter DC to all channels to obtain a deflection of the recording pen in the range of 5–10 mm. The technologist visually examines each calibration wave. As part of the calibration procedure, the technologist makes sure the equipment is properly plugged in, that all jacks are placed correctly, and that signal quality is adequate. Leads and sensors should be adjusted to control impedances and artifacts. Upon completion of the study, usually within 8 hours, the calibration procedure is repeated for 30 seconds, and results are compared with the initial calibration to ensure accuracy during the recording period.

Electrical Activity

Electrical activity is recorded by the polysomnogram (PSG) as tracings from three signal sources.

- Bioelectrical signals: These are generated by the patient's tissue and motion and recorded by surface electrodes to the display of the electroencephalogram, electrocardiogram, electrooculogram, and electromyogram.
- Transduced signals: These derive from sensors that convert action, such as chest wall movement, into electrical signals with the electrical signal generated by the sensor instead of the body.
- Equipment signals: Sometimes ancillary equipment, such as a carbon dioxide analyzer, is used during the PSG. This equipment, which has separate signal displays, outputs, and processing units, may be stand-alone or interfaced with the digital PSG equipment.

Physiological (Bio-) Calibrations

Electrocardiogram, Electroencephalogram, and Electrooculogram

Physiological (bio-) calibrations are performed by the technologist to evaluate signals generated by the patient.

- Electrocardiogram (ECG): The technologist checks the polarity of the reading to ensure the ECG tracing is not inverted, which is a sign that the jacks are inserted in incorrect channels.
- Electroencephalogram (EEG): The technologist asks the patient to relax with the eyes closed for 30 seconds or more, during which time the alpha waves on the EEG are typically prominent. Then the patient is asked to open the eyes for 30 seconds.
- Electrooculogram (EOG): When the patient is relaxed with the head still, the technologist asks the patient to look to the right and to the left a number of times, up and down a number of times, and finally to blink slowly about 5 times; the technologist then examines the EOG tracings to ensure that the three different types of eye movements are distinct on the recording.

Chin and Anterior Tibialis Electromyograms, Snore Sensor, Respiratory Sensors, and Airflow Sensors

Physiological (bio-) calibrations that must be completed before the polysomnogram (PSG) include:

- Chin electromyogram (cEMG): The technologist asks the patient to relax and remain quiet while determining that baseline muscle tone remains at 5 cm/amplitude or more. Then, the patient is asked to swallow, grit the teeth, and bite down to ensure that these actions show activity on the cEMG recording.
- Anterior tibialis electromyogram (atEMG): The technologist asks the patient to extend the legs and then to flex and extend the great toe on each foot, which should show activity on the atEMG tracings.
- Snore sensor: The technologist asks the patient to count to five out loud as this should cause deflection.
- Respiratory effort sensors and airflow sensors: The technologist asks the patient to stop breathing and hold the breath in briefly to ensure that the respiratory tracing shows a flat line. The patient is then asked to mimic paradoxical breathing by tightening and relaxing the thorax.

Physiological calibrations should be repeated at the end of the PSG to ensure that leads and sensors remain in the correct position and that recordings were accurate.

Frequency and Amplitude

Frequency and amplitude are waveforms that are recorded on polysomnography, using a standard time scale of 1 cm/sec. Frequency is the number of waves/cycles generated per second, and amplitude is the vertical height of a wave, determined by electrical voltage.

Machines are calibrated with a known signal so that waveforms can be interpreted according to height and sensitivity settings. The setting of 50 microvolts/cm, typically used for electroencephalograms, electrooculograms, chin electromyograms, and electromyograms, means that 50 microvolts of signal produce a standardized waveform that is 1 cm high. The wave height varies in relation to the sensitivity setting. While digital machines can record in a variety of ways, the data are displayed and recorded so that frequency and amplitude can be visually confirmed.

Filters

Filters are used to gain a more accurate recording by isolating bandwidths and reducing outside interference, such as from signals produced by the skin or muscle activity that causes artifacts. Most digital equipment records without the use of filters, but filters can later be applied to "clean up" the recording; however, filters (especially low frequency) can cause a phase shift that causes the wave to appear earlier or later. Filters are set in relation to the normal bandwidth of the test.

- Low-frequency filters eliminate signals below the normal bandwidth for a particular test.
- High-frequency filters eliminate signals above the normal bandwidth for a particular test.
- 60 Hz notch (band reject) filters remove signals (noise) produced in the
- 50–60 Hz range (power line interference) without affecting other frequencies, but this filter can interfere with recordings so it is rarely used except for anterior tibialis electromyograms.
- Band-pass filters record frequencies only within a particular range.

Frequency Settings

Frequency settings for filters vary, according to the test.

- Electroencephalogram (EEG) [standard sensitivity of 50 microvolts/cm]: Usually recorded in the range of 0.5–25 Hz, a low-frequency filter, therefore, would be set below the bottom range (at about 0.3), effectively reducing output below that level, and a high-frequency filter would be set above the top range (at 30–35 Hz), although when used to diagnose seizure activity, the high-frequency filter needs to be set higher (70–75 Hz) to allow for spiking during epileptic activity. Time constant is 0.25 seconds.
- Electrooculogram: Settings are similar to those for an EEG.
- Chin electromyogram (cEMG) and EMG: The low-frequency filters are typically set at 10 Hz, and the high-frequency filters are set at 90–100 Hz. Time constant is 0.1 seconds.
- Electrocardiogram (sensitivity at 1 millivolt/cm): The low-frequency filter is set at 1 Hz, and the high-frequency filters are set at 30–35 Hz. Time constant is 0.1 seconds.
- Respiratory sensors: The low-frequency filters are set at 0.1 Hz, and the high-frequency filters are set at 0.5 Hz. Time constant is 1 second.
- Oximetry (sensitivity at 1 volt/cm): The high-frequency filter is set at 15 Hz.

SAMPLING RATE

Sampling rates must be selected before testing when converting analog recordings to digital as they cannot be changed afterward in the way that filters can be changed. The converter uses predetermined intervals to assign a numeric value to waveforms. This value determines the amplitude (height) of the waveform. The sampling rate is equal to the number of sampled intervals done in 1 second. According to sampling theory, the minimum sampling rate is equal to at least twice the highest frequency sampled, but this will not provide an accurate representation of the analog waveform, so a higher sampling rate is necessary to achieve an adequate waveform. For example, sampling rates must be about 10 times higher for electroencephalograms (200–300 Hz with 30–35 Hz high-frequency settings) with adjustments if high-frequency filter settings are increased. Sampling rates should be selected for each channel.

WAVEFORM APPEARANCE

The appearance of the waveform is affected by filters. During calibration, when a 50-microvolt negative DC voltage is applied without filters, the waveform takes on a square appearance with an upward spike that is then sustained for the duration the voltage is applied. With low- and high-frequency filter settings, the shape and duration of waveforms alter as do the time constants, the difference between constant rise time and constant fall time:

- Rise time: Interval of time required for calibration waves to rise to 63% of amplitude.
- Fall time: Interval of time required for calibration waves to fall to 37% of amplitude.

Changing the setting of high- and low-frequency filters directly affects rise and fall time. Lowering the high-frequency filter setting increases rise time. Lowering the low-frequency filter setting increases fall time.

Documenting During Testing

EDS AND FATIGUE

Excessive daytime sleepiness (EDS), an increasing societal problem related to lack of adequate sleep, causes the patient to feel sleepy during waking hours to the point at which the person may fall asleep or feel the need to nap.
Fatigue, on the other hand, is a general feeling of tiredness, weakness, or lack of energy and may be related to physical or emotional problems. A person who is fatigued generally does not feel sleepy or have difficulty staying awake. Patients often do not distinguish between sleepiness and fatigue, so the technologist should question patients carefully to determine which they are experiencing:

- EDS: "Do you feel the need to sleep during the daytime?" "Do you feel drowsy?"
- Fatigue: "Do you feel as though you have no energy?" "Do you feel weary or weak?"

Sleepiness and fatigue scales may also be administered to help with diagnosis. Patients should evaluate sleepiness and fatigue at different times of the day with 9 am and 9 pm usually the time when people are most alert and 3 pm the least.

SUBJECTIVE SLEEPINESS EVALUATIONS

Subjective sleepiness evaluations, using various scales, are sometimes provided by the patient. While these evaluations are easy to use, take little time, and are usually available at no cost in print or online, the results should not be considered definitive because of a number of inherent weaknesses:

- Patients do not always report truthfully.
- Different scales measure different things and may not correlate.
- Some patients may receive a false positive and some a false negative.
- Scales are by their nature not objective so they are open to interpretation.
- The scales do not reflect comorbid conditions.
- People from different ethnic backgrounds may perceive sleep, sleepiness, and fatigue in different ways.
- Men and women may perceive sleep, sleepiness, and fatigue in different ways.

Stanford Sleepiness Scale

The Stanford Sleepiness Scale is a brief assessment used to determine if people have excessive daytime sleepiness (EDS). The scale is used at a number of different times during the day as people may report feeling sleepy at different times, especially in the late afternoon, a low period of alertness for most people. The scale lists seven descriptors that rate increasing levels of sleepiness. People with an EDS score of 4–7 have a sleep debt that interferes with functioning:

Fully alert and awake	1
Functioning and concentrating well but slightly sluggish.	2
Awake and functioning but not fully alert	3
Slightly foggy	4
Foggy, slightly drowsy	5
Feeling sleepy and drowsy and having difficulty staying awake	6
Nearing onset of sleep and awake dreaming	7
Sleeping	X

Epworth Sleepiness Scale

The Epworth Sleepiness Scale evaluates how likely a person is to fall asleep during a number of different activities. The person rates each situation on a scale of 0–3, corresponding to the chance of falling asleep (none, slight, moderate, or high). Situations queried include the following:

- Sitting and reading
- Watching television
- Sitting quietly in a public place, such as a meeting, movie, or theater
- Sitting as a passenger in a car for an hour or more with no break
- Lying down for an afternoon rest
- Sitting and visiting with someone
- Sitting quietly after eating lunch (which did not include alcohol)
- Sitting in a car while stopped in traffic for a few minutes

Scores are totaled with 1–6 indicating the person is receiving adequate sleep. The average score for most people is 7–8, but scores of 9 or higher indicate the person has a high index for sleepiness and should have further testing.

Sleep–Wake Activity Inventory

The Sleep-Wake Activity Inventory (SWAI) is a comprehensive instrument that includes subscales that measure a number of different aspects of sleep disorders: excessive daytime sleepiness (EDS), nocturnal sleep, relaxing ability, energy, social desirability, and psychological distress. The EDS subscale asks the patient to score nine different statements about sleepiness on 1–9 scale (always present to never present). Descriptors include:

- I fall asleep while watching television.
- I am able to nap anywhere.
- I fall asleep in the middle of a conversation.
- I feel drowsy within a few minutes while driving.
- I feel drowsy within 10 minutes of sitting quietly.
- I fall asleep during visits with friends.
- I feel sleepy after 15 minutes of reading.
- I fall asleep when I am relaxed.
- I fall asleep when I am riding in a car as a passenger.

Scores are added together. A score 50 or more is normal, but 40–50 suggests sleepiness, and a score of 40 or less indicates EDS.

Fatigue Severity Scale

The Fatigue Severity Scale contains a list of nine descriptions related to fatigue. The patient scores each statement on a 1–7 scale (strongly disagree to strongly agree). Descriptors include:

- I have less motivation when I am fatigued.
- I become fatigued when I exercise.
- I become fatigued easily.
- My fatigue interferes with my ability to function physically.
- I experience frequent problems because of fatigue.
- I cannot carry out sustained physical activities/functioning because of fatigue.
- I cannot adequately carry out all of my duties and responsibilities because of fatigue.
- Fatigue is one of the three most disabling symptoms that I experience.
- My work, social, and family life suffer because of my fatigue.

The scores are added together with scores of 9–35 in the normal range and scores above 35 suggesting a high degree of fatigue.

Recording

Documenting observations of the patient during the polysomnogram (PSG) (even if video monitoring is used) is very important so that an accurate sleep study report can be generated at the end of the procedure as not all pertinent information is obvious from the data generated. The following must be documented:

- Time lights go out and lights go on
- Total recording time
- Patient's emotional status, including anxiety or confusion that may impact results
- Patient's physical status, including unusual motor activity and nocturia
- Patient's position (supine, head elevated, sitting)
- Descriptions of breathing/snoring or other audible sounds
- Atypical findings, such as REM sleep behavior disorder

The technologist should not rely on memory but should note unusual events as they occur, marking the time, duration, and frequency, so that the events can be correlated with the recordings.

Sleep Technologist's Interventions

Sleep technologist's interventions that occur during the polysomnogram, including application of electrodes and sensors, calibrations, and physiological calibrations, must be documented. Documentation should include a description of the event, the exact time of onset, duration of time, and time event ends. Important information to document includes:

- Reattachment of dislodged electrodes and sensors
- Assisting patient to change positions
- Diaper changes and episodes of incontinence or nocturia
- Patient requests (e.g., water, change in temperature, need for extra blankets)
- Patient or parent complaints (e.g., discomfort, anxiety, fear)
- Parasomnias (e.g., sleepwalking, talking in sleep, unusual motor activity)
- Parent or caregiver interventions (e.g., comforting a frightened child, nursing or feeding an infant)
- Arousals
- Patient behaviors relevant to artifacts in recordings
- Evidence of seizures

Identifying and Responding to Data Issues

Artifacts

Artifacts, extraneous signals, are common during polysomnography; some relate to normal activity, such as muscle movement or snoring. The technologist must monitor, identify, and correct artifacts as necessary by:

- Checking other channels to determine if the artifacts are occurring in only one channel or adjacent channels as well. If in only one channel, then the artifact may be related to a single lead.
- Determining if the affected channels share a reference lead as this suggests the artifact relates to the reference.
- Changing the derivation of the input signal, typically to the opposite side, so if C4 shows artifacts, change to C3.
- Monitoring constantly and change derivations as needed through system referencing or the use of multiple channels.

Physiological Artifacts

Physiological artifacts can be caused by numerous factors (extraneous signals) that alter the results of polysomnography.

Cause	Result	Correction
Muscle (electromyogram EMG)	The background electroencephalogram (EEG) or electro-oculogram may be obscured and other signals distorted, depending on the type of muscle activity.	Encourage patient to relax, deep breathe, and slightly open the jaw to reduce tension. Report on visual observations when artifacts occur, noting signs of seizures or a sleep behavior disorder. Ensure electrodes are correctly attached.

Cause	Result	Correction
Skin, irritation (rash)	Irritation, such as a skin rash, can alter the skin's electrical signal, causing high impedance.	Place electrode in a different area, avoiding irritated skin.
Vibration	Leg movement or snoring can cause high-frequency artifacts.	Note and record all artifacts; correction is not usually possible.
Perspiration (EEG)	Excess perspiration may cause slow-frequency artifacts or can be similar to delta waves (high frequency).	Cool patient by changing room temperature or using fans.
Swallow (EEG)	Swallowing can result in slow waves in temporal areas, typical on arousal.	Note and record; correction not usually possible.
Retinal disease (EOG)	The affected eye may interfere with electrical signal.	Note activity of unaffected eye, or use other measures.
Artificial eye (EOG)	The prosthetic eye does not generate electrical signals.	Note underlying frontal EEG activity.
Blink (EOG)	Produces slow waves, depending on type and speed of activity.	Note and record; correction not usually possible.
Eye muscle abnormality (weakness, hyperactivity, paralysis) [EOG, EEG]	Abnormalities may alter EOG readings, depending on the type of abnormality. Rectus movement can cause spike in EEG (frontotemporal).	Note activity of unaffected eye or use other measures.

Abbreviations: EEG = electroencephalogram; and EOG = electrooculogram.

Mechanical Artifacts

Mechanical artifacts relate to interference caused by the equipment.

Cause	Result	Correction
ECG in EEG, EOG, or EMG channels	ECG tracing appears in other channels.	Re-reference (double reference) channels for EEG/EOG to reference leads A_1 and A_2. Ensure electrodes are correctly placed and attached. Avoid applying reference electrodes to fat, soft tissue. Use common mode rejection for EMG artifacts, or reattach EMG electrodes.
Electrode pop (sharp, spiking deflection)	Electrode pops are generally related to only one electrode but may be observed in multiple channels.	Remove, reprep skin, and reattach electrode. Pops may result from pressure on electrodes, dirty electrodes, or loose wires.
Cardio-ballistic (sensors)	Sensors (respiratory effort, airflow) pick up pulse waves from ECG.	Note and record; correction not usually possible.

Mechanical artifacts can result from problems with equipment, including incorrect application or dislodging of electrodes and sensors.

Cause	Result	Correction
Condensation in CPAP tubing.	Fluid in tubing can cause M-shaped waveform in airflow channel.	Remove fluid from tubing.
Loose belt (sensors)	Tracings are flat despite evidence of movement or respirations.	Reapply belt correctly.
Misplacement of airflow sensor	Sensor does not record changes in temperature/airflow.	Reposition.
Electrodes, loose or improperly secured	High-frequency noise combined with high amplitude can slow activity.	Remove, reprep skin, and reattach electrode.
Oximetry channel	Inaccurate recordings of oxygen saturation can result from improperly attached oximeter.	Check placement and ensure fingernail is free of polish.

Abbreviations: ECG = electrocardiogram; EEG = electroencephalogram; EOG = electrooculogram; EMG = electromyogram; and CPAP = continuous positive airway pressure.

Recording-Related Artifacts

Recording-related artifacts may relate to choice of channels or filters as well as interference from equipment.

Cause	Result	Correction
50–60 Hz	Caused by poor grounding of EEG electrodes or interference from electrical leakage from other equipment; 50–60 Hz artifacts can occur in EMG channels, especially leg EMGs.	Use common mode rejection. A 50–60 notch filter may remove artifacts at 50–60 Hz, but do not use in EEG or EOG channels as artifacts there usually indicate improper connection.
Multiple channel recordings	Multiple source artifacts can make a recording unreadable, and multiple channels cannot be shown at the same time so important data may be missed.	Reconsider approach.
Excessive filtering	Filtering can distort data and mask problems that require correction.	Avoid using filters to reduce artifacts, and do not use filters to remove artifacts unless underlying physiological signals are adequate.

Abbreviations: EEG = electroencephalogram; EMG = electromyogram; and EOG = electrooculogram.

Multiple Sleep Latency Tests

The multiple sleep latency test (MSLT) measures sleepiness during waking hours and the tendency of a person to fall asleep. The MSLT may diagnose narcolepsy and idiopathic hypersomnia and determine the effectiveness of therapy. Elements include:

- Patient keeps a 2-week sleep diary before testing, sometimes with actigraphy, to identify sleeping patterns.
- Medications are assessed and withheld when possible if they affect sleep. Stimulants should be discontinued for 2 weeks before testing.

- The MSLT must be preceded by nocturnal polysomnography, and the montage includes electroencephalogram, electrooculogram, chin electromyogram, and electrocardiogram.
- MSLT includes five nap periods with first within 3 hours of a nocturnal polysomnogram and then spaced at 2 hours after start of preceding nap.
- Patients report their subjective evaluation of sleepiness 45 minutes before five designated nap periods, and physiological calibrations are done 5 minutes before onset of nap period.
- No smoking is allowed within 30 minutes of starting a nap and no strenuous activity within 15 minutes.
- Mean sleep latency is evaluated.

Maintenance of Wakefulness Test

The maintenance of wakefulness test (MWT), done to assess sleepiness and effectiveness of treatment, determines the patient's ability to stay awake in the daytime. The MWT may be done with the multiple sleep latency test (MSLT). Elements include:

- A 2-week sleep diary and nocturnal polysomnogram may be done before the MWT, depending on the patient.
- Montage is similar to the MSLT: electroencephalogram, electrooculogram, chin electromyogram, and electrocardiogram.
- Patient is placed at rest, sitting in bed with low lights for four 40-minute periods, spaced at 2 hours, and advised to remain awake but not to engage in activities (e.g., singing, moving).
- Sleep latency (onset of sleep) is measured with fewer than 8 minutes considered abnormal. About half of normal sleepers remain awake during all 40-minute periods.
- Patient is awakened 90 seconds after falling asleep as duration of sleep is not important for the MWT alone.
- If the patient does not fall asleep during the 40-minute resting period, the test is terminated.

Wrist Actigraphy

Wrist actigraphy uses a portable device worn on the wrist that records and analyzes movement. Information stored in the device is downloaded into a computer. A number of different devices are available, and they evaluate movement in different ways, using a single channel, so determining the validity of the reports or comparing it to standard polysomnography is problematic, especially if patients have movement disorders or periods of quiet (without moving) during waking hours. Because of these limitations, wrist actigraphy should be used for multiple days (at least three 24-hour periods with up to 7 days optimal) to help to identify patterns of sleep/waking. Wrist actigraphy alone is not usually adequate for diagnosis of sleep disordered breathing or periodic limb movement but can be used to evaluate other sleep disorders. The patient should keep a diary of activities during wrist actigraphy to identify artifacts and to aid in interpretation of the results. Scoring varies, according to the manufacturer's guidelines.

Infant Polysomnograms

Infant polysomnograms (PSGs) may be done for short (between feedings) or extended (overnight) periods, but short examinations may not render adequate information, so longer testing is recommended. Some modifications are necessary for infant PSGs. Usually a parent or caregiver remains in the room with the infant although the person should be advised not to disturb the child except for feeding and diaper changes during the test. For toddlers, the room should be as child friendly as possible. The temperature is usually maintained at about 23°C, and the child should be in a crib or secure bed with side rails. Using play and dolls to show placement of electrodes may be helpful for small children. Safety measures should be in place to secure all electrical outlets, supplies, and equipment.

Placing Electrodes and Sensors for Infant/Child Polysomnograms

Infant/child polysomnograms (PSGs) may require some modification when placing electrodes and sensors. Parents may hold or soothe the child when leads are applied. There are a number of factors to consider:

- Collodion may cause eye irritation, so paste or other adhesive may be used. Pasted electrodes increase slow-frequency electroencephalogram (EEG) artifacts, reduced by increasing a low-frequency filter to 1 Hz (but this will interfere with slow-wave EEG activity).
- Toddlers may require a gauze turban or cap to keep scalp electrodes in place.
- Infants may need their hands covered with socks, and toddlers may need parents to prevent the child from touching leads until the child is asleep.
- Bundling and taping of leads can prevent dislodgement.
- Re-referencing/re-montaging may be necessary if children are active.
- Higher sampling rates are needed to detect seizure activity (EEG ≥ 500 Hz and electrooculogram/electromyogram ≥ 200 Hz).
- A chin electromyogram should be placed where it will not come in contact with drool.
- Respiratory effort belts and sensors may need to be secured with tape.

PH Ssensor

A pH sensor may be placed in the esophagus to diagnose gastric acid reflux in infants and children. In infants, a thin wire with a sensor at the end is passed nasally, but older children (or adults) may be able to swallow the sensor with fluids. There are two types of sensors that are used:

- Antimony/antimony oxide electrode: The small pellet-like sensor is antimony coated with antimony oxide. A skin reference electrode is needed for this type.
- Glass electrode: The glass electrode is a combined sensor and reference electrode (2–4 mm diameter). It is inserted into the esophagus in the same manner as the antimony/antimony oxide electrode. The glass electrode has a high level of electrical impedance that can interfere with readings and can be broken if not handled properly, although it is unlikely to break when positioned in the esophagus.

Infant Polysomnogram, Sensors and Oximeter

Sensors for the infant polysomnogram must be placed carefully to ensure accurate recording.

- Respiratory effort sensors: It is important that the sensors (inductance plethysmography or piezo crystal bands) are the correct size and secured with tape if necessary. The thoracic band is placed immediately above the nipple and the abdominal band, about the umbilicus.
- Position sensor: This sensor is placed according to the manufacturer's directions, usually on the lower back (over the diaper) with the infant in the supine position.
- Motion sensor: This sensor is placed on a limb, which is moved to ensure that the signal is adequate.

The oximeter is placed carefully on the hand or foot of the infant, and secured with wrapping as necessary, avoiding excess padding that might increase heat and affect readings.

Interventions During Infant Polysomnogram

Interventions during an infant polysomnogram are made as indicated by what the technologist observes. Emergency action may be needed if an infant has apneic periods for over 20 seconds:

- The oxygen saturation and heart rate are noted to determine if the infant is showing a decrease, but no intervention is necessary until the oxygen saturation level is less than 85% or the heart rate is less than 60 for 10 seconds. When oxygen saturation and heart rate have fallen to the critical points, intervention is indicated:
- The infant is stimulated by flicking the thumb against the heels or the bottom of the feet.
- If there is no improvement, the airway and position are checked, using suction to clear airways if necessary. Oxygen per bag is provided; a few puffs are administered and continued until oxygen saturation and heart rate return to normal.
- If the infant's condition still does not improve, emergency procedures are followed (a code is called for a physician).
- The electroencephalogram is checked for indications of seizure activity.

American Academy of Pediatrics Clinical Guidelines for OSAS

The American Academy of Pediatrics has issued clinical guidelines for the diagnosis and treatment of obstructive sleep apnea syndrome (OSAS). Recommendations include:

- All children are screened for snoring, observed apnea, restlessness during sleep, daytime sleepiness, or neurobehavioral abnormalities.
- Physical exam notes abnormalities that may relate to OSAS.
- If indications of OSAS are present:
  - High-risk children with co-morbid conditions should be immediately referred to a specialist.
  - Children who are not high risk but show evidence of cardiac or respiratory failure should have further evaluation in consultation with a specialist.
  - Children who are not high risk and do not show evidence of cardiac or respiratory failure should be referred for polysomnography to diagnose OSAS.
- Tonsillectomy/adenoidectomy is the first-line treatment for OSAS with continuous positive airway pressure an option for those unable to have surgery or for those who do not respond to surgical treatment.
- High-risk children should be monitored as inpatients after surgery.
- Re-evaluation is needed after surgery to determine effectiveness.

American Thoracic Society, Standards/Indications for Cardiopulmonary Sleep Studies in Children

General Guidelines

The American Thoracic Society issued standards and indications for pediatric cardiopulmonary sleep studies to assist with the diagnosis of sleep-related breathing disorders (e.g., obstructive sleep apnea syndrome, OSAS) in children. Indications for polysomnography include:

- Differentiating benign snoring or primary snoring from pathological snoring that involves periods of apnea.
- Evaluating children who experience disturbances in patterns of sleep, including waking sleepiness, who fail to thrive, or who exhibit cor pulmonale or polycythemia, especially in children who snore.
- Clarifying clinical observations and diagnosis.

- Evaluating children with laryngomalacia and stridor (worsening at night).
- Evaluating the effects of obesity if other symptoms, such as snoring, sleep disturbance, or hypercapnia, are present.
- Evaluating the condition of the child with sickle cell disease with evidence of OSAS or veno-occlusive disease.
- Noting progress after treatment (4 weeks postsurgical) or weight loss (if indicated to control OSAS).
- Administering the multiple sleep latency test to evaluate excessive daytime sleepiness if OSAS is not noted.
- Assisting with titrating continuous positive airway pressure in those with OSAS.

Bronchopulmonary Dysplasia and Cystic Fibrosis

The American Thoracic Society has established recommendations regarding polysomnography for a number of childhood disorders.

Broncho-pulmonary dysplasia	Children may receive supplemental oxygen to maintain oxygen saturation at more than 92%.
	Assess oxygen saturation levels during both waking and sleeping hours to determine if hypoxemia occurs. Assess oxygen saturation levels after oxygen is discontinued if unexplained symptoms occur, such as cor pulmonale, polycythemia, and failure to thrive. Evaluate bradycardia occurring without apnea and snoring or suspected upper airway obstruction. Evaluate gastric reflux disease (pH sensor).
Cystic fibrosis	Oxygen desaturation may occur without apnea.
	Provide continuous nocturnal oximetry if daytime oxygen saturation level is less than 95%.
	Use nocturnal oximetry for at least 8 hours if child has headaches in the morning, cor pulmonale, polycythemia, or daytime sleepiness. Diagnose OSAS in a child receiving supplemental oxygen with symptoms of cor pulmonale, polycythemia, and decrease in nocturnal oxygen saturation.
	Determine adverse effects of supplemental oxygen in the presence of severe lung disease.

Asthma and Neuromuscular Disorders

The American Thoracic Society has established recommendations for polysomnography for a number of childhood disorders.

Asthma	Do a polysomnography with pH sensor if nocturnal symptoms may be related to gastroesophageal reflux disease.
	Use nocturnal oximetry for children who experience asthma attacks during the night, complain of headaches on awakening, or have other types of disturbed sleep or cor pulmonale.

Neuro-muscular disorders (e.g., muscular dystrophy, cerebral palsy)	Do a polysomnography with end-tidal or transcutaneous carbon dioxide monitoring: If respiratory muscles are weak and forced vital capacity is less than 40%, PIP is less than 15 cm H_2O, snoring is evident, or child has difficulty swallowing. If impairment is beyond that expected by diagnosis occurs, including snoring, cor pulmonale, headache on awakening, failure to thrive, and delay in development. As part of planning for nocturnal mechanical ventilation. For evaluation of respiratory treatment and care. As preoperative or postoperative assessment.

Alveolar Hypoventilation Syndrome and Infantile Apnea/Bradycardia

The American Thoracic Society has established recommendations for polysomnography for a number of childhood disorders.

Alveolar hypoventilation syndrome	Polysomnography with carbon dioxide monitoring is indicated: To determine severity of disorder. To evaluate condition/treatment (periodically). To evaluate clinically unstable children with symptoms that include cor pulmonale, polycythemia, failure to thrive, developmental delay, headaches upon awakening, or altered mental status.
Infantile apnea/ bradycardia	While polysomnography is not recommended for routine evaluation of infants with apnea/bradycardia experiencing an apparent life-threatening event, it may be indicated: To clarify the frequency of apnea and type and alterations in the EEG, ECG and other parameters, especially if OSAS or ineffective control of respiration is suspected or bradycardia occurs without central apnea.

Abbreviations: EEG = electroencephalogram, ECG = electrocardiogram; and OSAS = obstructive sleep apnea syndrome.

Identifying and Responding to Patient Needs

Nonrespiratory Conditions That Impact Sleep in Infants and Small Children

Nonrespiratory physical conditions can often impact the sleep of infants and young children.

Neonates and infants	Colic is a circadian disorder in which the child develops abdominal cramping and pain during the evening and night.
	Gastric reflux or milk intolerance also can result in crying and discomfort but usually is also evident during the daytime.
	CSA and OSA may result in crying at night.
Ages 1–5	Non-REM parasomnias may occur.
	The child may have reduced sleeping needs for both nighttime sleeping and napping, and this can lead to frustration and resistance to sleeping that results in sleeping disorders, such as conditioned insomnia.
	The child may experience sleep terrors, nightmares, or nocturnal seizures that interfere with sleep.

Abbreviations: CSA = central sleep apnea; and OSA = obstructive sleep apnea.

Nonrespiratory Conditions Impacting Sleep in School-Age Children and Adolescents

Nonrespiratory physical conditions can often impact the sleep of school-age and adolescent children.

Ages 5–11	Non-REM parasomnias may occur.
	The child may be sensitive to noise and arouse easily.
	Sleep hygiene may be inadequate.
	The child may experience exaggerated fears (e.g., loss of parent, injury) that interfere with sleep.
Adolescents	Medications used to treat behavioral/psychiatric disorders may interfere with sleep.
	Busy schedules often preclude adequate sleep.
	Delayed sleep phase is common, so the adolescent goes to sleep later and has difficulty awakening because of inadequate total sleep time.
	Onset of narcolepsy may occur during adolescence.

Sleep Requirements for Infants

Sleep requirements for infants include:

0–1 months	The newborn sleeps about 16.5 hr/d, evenly spaced through both day and night.
2–4 months	The infant continues to sleep a lot, about 15 hr/d but is often awake for periods in the morning, afternoon, and evening, so sleeping time during the night exceeds sleep time during the daytime by about an hour.
4–6 months	The child sleeps about 10–11 hours at night with two to three daytime naps that total 3–4 hours with total sleep time of 14.25 hours.
6–8 months	The child begins to have more waking hours, sleeping 10–11 hours with two naps and total sleep time of about 14–14.25 hours.
8–10 months	The child continues to sleep about 10–11 hours at night and usually sleeps through the night, with two naps in the daytime and total sleep time of about 14 hours.
10–12 months	The child continues to sleep 10–11 hours at night with two naps in the daytime with total sleep time of about 13.75 hours.

Sleep Requirements for Children

Sleep requirements for children slowly decrease as they eliminate daytime naps and become more engaged in activities.

1–2 years	As the infant becomes more active, the nighttime requirements remain at 10.75 hours, but daytime sleeping of two naps decreases in duration to 2–3 hours for a total of 13 hours sleep by age 2.
3–4 years	During this transitional stage, the child's nighttime sleeping time increases slightly as the daytime nap is eliminated, so those napping sleep a total of 10.25 hours during the night (plus a daytime nap), increasing to 11.50 hours when naps cease.

5–8 years	The child is more active, and the schedule is more regimented, precluding naps, as the child attends school with overall sleeping time decreasing from 11 hours total at 5 years to 10.25 hours at 8 years.
9–11 years	As the child becomes more engaged in activities, total sleep time slowly decreases from 10 hours at age 9 to 9.5 hours by age 11.

Sleep Requirements for Adolescents

Sleep requirements for adolescents remain relatively high during early adolescence but decrease to adult levels by age 18. Because children mature at different rates, not all children will have the same requirements at the same age. Girls tend to mature earlier than boys, and this can impact their sleep requirements:

11–14 years	This is a transitional time for children as their hormones and their bodies go through changes that may increase anxiety and impact sleep time. Children mature at varying rates, so there are wide differences with total sleeping hours usually ranging from 9.5 to 9 hours.
15–18 years	As the child begins to mature into an adult, he or she may engage in activities that impact sleep, but sleeping requirements range from 8.75 hours at age 15 to 8.25 hours at age 18.

Infant/Child Polysomnography

During infant/child polysomnography, close observation of children is necessary to relate activities to recorded data, as this information may be critical in developing a diagnosis for sleep-related disorders.

Newborn to 5 years	The lab tries to emulate the sleep environment and activities of the child's home as much as possible, and the technologist observes the behaviors of both the child and parents, including interactions and bedtime rituals.
5–12 years	The technologist reviews the child's sleep log or parental report of the child's sleeping habits and carefully notes behaviors, such as stalling or tantrums that may delay bedtime. The child's ability to initiate sleep should be observed as well as episodes of fidgeting, restlessness, or crying. Bedtime habits or rituals (e.g., reading, watching television, co-sleeping) are followed and documented as they may affect sleep onset.
12–18 years	While observations are similar to those of adults, adolescents often are concerned about privacy and may feel uncomfortable sleeping under the observation of a technologist of the opposite gender; thus, a frank discussion that allows the adolescent to express opinions is important.

Neuromuscular Diseases

Spinal Cord Injury

Neuromuscular diseases can impair respiratory muscles, including pharyngeal, intercostal, and diaphragm muscles, resulting in the increased risk of obstructive sleep apnea as well as aspiration during sleep and hypoventilation. The polysomnogram (PSG) aids in determining respiratory impairment and the need for assisted ventilation.

Spinal cord injury	Impairment relates to the level of the injury.
	C4 and higher: Complete paralysis of muscles of respiration (i.e., intercostal, diaphragmatic, abdominal), so the patient requires a ventilator.
	C4–T6: Varying degrees of muscle weakness and paralysis, so even though the person does not require a ventilator, respirations may not be adequate.
	T6–T12: Allows for normal breathing, but the muscles that control cough are impaired.
	Below T12: Does not affect muscles related to respirations or coughing.
	The PSG assesses the patient for hypoventi-lation and hypoxia.

Spina Bifida and Myelomeningocele

Spina bifida is a neural tube defect with an incomplete spinal cord and often missing vertebrae that allow the meninges and spinal cord to protrude through the opening.
Myelomeningocele is a spina bifida cystica with the meningeal sac containing spinal fluid and part of the spinal cord and nerves, resulting in varying degrees of muscle paralysis and loss of sensation below the area of involvement as well as hydrocephalus. Children are at increased risk for apnea (especially obstructive sleep apnea and central sleep apnea), hypoventilation, and aspiration. The nocturnal polysomnogram is important as patterns of hypoventilation and sleep-disordered breathing may not be obvious during waking hours. Infants with myelomeningocele are less likely to arouse in response to hypercapnia than other infants.

Pseudohypertrophic Duchenne Muscular Dystrophy

Pseudohypertrophic Duchenne muscular dystrophy is the most common form of muscular dystrophy. Pseudohypertrophic refers to enlargement of the muscles by fatty infiltration associated with muscular atrophy, which causes contractures and deformities of joints and abnormal skeletal development, such as scoliosis, that can impair breathing. As the disease progresses, it involves the muscles of the diaphragm and other muscles, such as the oropharyngeal, which are needed for respiration. Sleep-disordered breathing may be obvious during polysomnography even though pulmonary function tests are normal during waking hours. Typical sleep-related problems include the following:

- Increasing sleep disruption
- Decrease in vital capacity to less than 2 L
- Obstructive sleep apnea
- Hypercapnia and oxygen desaturation during REM sleep, progressing to non-REM sleep as the condition worsens
- Children whose disease has progressed may require ventilatory support.

Spinal Muscular Atrophy

Spinal muscular atrophy (SMA) comprises a number of different neuromuscular diseases with type I (Werdnig-Hoffman disease or "floppy infant syndrome") the most severe with progressive weakness and wasting of skeletal muscles caused by degeneration of anterior horn cells of the spinal cord and the motor nuclei of the brainstem. Children with type I are typically hypotonic at birth and are prone to aspiration because of weakness of the intercostal muscles, although the diaphragm is usually unaffected. These children may have frequent aspirations and pneumonia.

Polysomnography may show hypoventilation, sleep apnea, and hypoxemia. Types II and III are characterized by weakness of peripheral muscles and scoliosis. Respiratory muscles may also have some degree of weakness, leading to respiratory failure. With SMA, polysomnography may indicate hypoventilation and hypoxemia, suggesting the need for noninvasive ventilation to prevent or delay progression of respiratory failure.

Congenital Myotonic Dystrophy

Congenital myotonic dystrophy causes damage during the fetal period that results in hypoplasia of the lungs and diaphragm; thus, the infant requires ventilatory support at birth. Both apnea and sleep-disordered breathing may occur in the neonatal period, and nocturnal hypoventilation may persist. Symptoms vary, depending on the severity of the disease, with some children exhibiting only slight hypotonia and impaired sucking and swallowing reflexes (increasing the risk of aspiration), while others present with severe respiratory failure. Older children and adolescents may have hypersomnolence, obstructive sleep apnea, and disruption of sleep as well as gastroesophageal reflux, so a polysomnogram may require a pH sensor. Cardiac arrhythmias are common and may be associated with hypercapnia, hypoxemia, and hypoventilation (resulting in acidosis), so careful observation of the electrocardiogram tracings is critical.

Infant and Pediatric Polysomnography and Neuromuscular Diseases

Infant and pediatric polysomnography is an essential component of evaluation of children with neuromuscular diseases to determine cardiorespiratory impairment and to establish the need for assisted ventilation during sleep because impaired sleeping/ventilation increases the risk of respiratory failure. Polysomnography should be done as soon after diagnosis as possible to establish baseline readings, followed by periodic polysomnography to note the progress of the disease. Because of the child's impaired sensation or ability to move, care must be taken during the polysomnogram to prevent injury or irritation.

- Lifts are available to assist in moving older children.
- The child's body is positioned with adequate cushioning and support, using pillows or bolsters, making sure to maintain proper body alignment.
- Linens must be kept smooth and free of wrinkles.
- The child must be turned and moved carefully, avoiding jerking.

Montage Requirements for Children with Neuromuscular Diseases

Montage requirements for children with neuromuscular diseases are listed below.

EEG, EOG, and cEMG	Sleep staging shows progression of disease.
	Mild: Frequent arousal and decreased REM and stage 1 non-REM sleep
	Moderate: Frequent arousals and awakening and deceased REM sleep
	Advanced: Short arousal and awakening after prolonged periods of desaturation and absent REM sleep
Oximetry	Mild: ≤ 96%
	Moderate: ⍰ 94% with desaturation during REM sleep
	Advanced: ⍰ 92% with desaturation during REM and non-REM sleep
Respiratory effort	Respiratory effort varies with the type of disorder and the degree of muscle impairment; thus, it may be difficult to judge respiratory effort. Inductance plethysmography is most accurate.
Airflow	Mild: Respiratory rate is increased.
	Moderate: Respiratory rate is normal to increased.

	Advanced: Respiratory rate is normal.
	Snoring may indicate obstruction.
$etCO_2$ continue transition monitoring.	Mild: < 45 torr
	Moderate: ⍰ 45 torr
	Advanced: ⍰ 50 torr
	Increases may be evident before oxygen desaturation with onset of hypoventilation.
ECG	Cardiac arrhythmias are common with neuromuscular diseases.
Video	Correlating activity with recordings is essential.

Abbreviations: EEG = electroencephalogram; EOG = electrooculogram; cEMG = chin electromyogram; ECG = electrocardiogram; and $etCO_2$ = end-tidal carbon dioxide.

Noninvasive Ventilation

Noninvasive ventilation (NIV) is used with patients with neuromuscular disease to prevent or delay respiratory failure and the use of more invasive ventilatory measures; however, in some cases, such as Duchenne's muscular dystrophy, too early use of NIV may worsen respiratory failure. NIV may be implemented during polysomnography. Factors to consider include:

- Gas exchange goals: This includes acceptable oxygen saturation and carbon dioxide levels and parameters for use. The physician's orders should explicitly state the levels at which NIV is to be implemented.
- Type of ventilation, device, and settings.
- Accessibility of a physician in case of emergencies.
- Interface: The oronasal mask must be used with care for neuromuscular patients because they cannot easily remove the mask. Nasal prongs may not be an appropriate fit for small children and may not provide adequate ventilation.

Physiological Effects of Sleep

The physiological effects of sleep must be considered with children with pulmonary disorders because sleep can exacerbate respiratory problems.

- Reduced tidal volume resulting in reduced lung volume and minute ventilation
- Reduced functional residual volume (and reduced store of oxygen), resulting from hypotonia of respiratory muscles (primarily during REM sleep), displacement of the diaphragm (cephalad), central pooling of blood, and increased elasticity of lungs
- Increased chest wall compliance from muscle hypotonia
- Increased airway resistance
- Decreased basal metabolic rate, resulting in decreased production of carbon dioxide counterbalanced by a simultaneous decrease in alveolar ventilation that results in an overall increase in carbon dioxide by 5–6 torr above normal value
- Decreased central nervous system response to chemical changes (e.g., hypoxia, hypercapnia) or mechanical changes (e.g., respirations), resulting in reduced respiratory drive (again increasing carbon dioxide), especially during REM sleep
- Altered arousal threshold

Proper Body Mechanics

Proper body mechanics must be used by sleep technicians to prevent back injury when assisting patients to change position during the night. If a patient falls, the technician should not attempt to lift the patient back into bed but should call for assistance; the patient must be examined for injuries and lifted safely. Lifting techniques include the following:

- Avoid bending at the waist to lift or reach for items. Stoop down with the knees bent.
- Avoid stretching overhead to reach for items on high shelves or out of reach. Use a step stool or grip tool with extension.
- Avoid pushing or pulling with the arms. Use the whole body to relieve strain on the arms and back.
- Avoid reaching, bending, or twisting to lift. Stand close to the person or item to be lifted, bend knees and hips, and use the muscles in the legs to support weight rather than the back or arms.

Thermoregulation

Thermoregulation involves systems that are controlled automatically with the exception of engaging in physical activity and sleeping. The normal body temperature is about 37°C, but this varies about 1°, according to the circadian cycle and activities, with low points at about 3 am and high points at 6 pm. People who suffer sleep deprivation tend to maintain a higher temperature in the morning with less overall variation. Body heat dissipates through conduction, convection, radiation, and evaporation. The body retains or increases heat though shivering, muscle activity, changes in hormones, changes in posture, vasoconstriction, and environmental changes (increased temperature, clothing). Thermoregulation is less stable in older adults. Production of heat decreases, and heat loss increases. The temperature-regulating mechanism of the hypothalamus may reset internal temperature control at a lower level. Infants and children have larger body surface-to-weight ratios than adults, thinner skin, and a lower fat content. Infants can only produce heat by activity, shivering (> 3 months of age), and nonshivering thermogenesis.

Sleep Deprivation

Sleep deprivation is becoming more common as many adults as well as teenagers and some children sleep less than 7 hours a night. Short-term sleep deprivation (1–2 days) seems to have no long-lasting effects, but long-term sleep deprivation can cause some of the following harmful effects:

- Changes in thermoregulation
- Emotional lability
- Increased stress and increased response to stress
- Increased blood pressure
- Impaired functioning
- Increased risk of accidents (e.g., auto, machinery, falls)
- Chronic sleepiness and fatigue

When sleep deprivation is chronic, people often are unable to judge their degree of sleepiness, using common tests, such as the Stanford Sleepiness Scale, so subjective reports may not indicate the actual degree of sleepiness. The Epworth Sleepiness Scale is usually more accurate. Sleep deprivation may be related to poor health, medications, and lifestyle choices.

Stress and Anxiety and the Sympathetic Nervous System

The sympathetic nervous system turns on the physiologic response to stress and anxiety and readies the body to react. The hypothalamus stimulates the pituitary gland to secrete a hormone, leading to increased cortisol levels. The sympathetic nervous system usually leads to a decrease in blood flow in the gastrointestinal tract. This decreases appetite and movement of the intestinal tract. The neuromuscular system is charged up and ready to respond. Reflex time is increased, and there can be some twitching or shaking of muscles. The need for sleep is greatly reduced, leading to periods of insomnia. The facial expression may be tense and anxious, and the individual may actually pace about. The individual may have uncontrolled muscle movements, restlessness, and fast speech and may startle easily. The skin may become flushed or itchy with increased sweat gland production.

Stress and Anxiety and the Parasympathetic Nervous System

The parasympathetic nervous system can activate in some individuals during stress, although usually individuals respond to stress and anxiety by activation of the sympathetic nervous system, which puts the body in a state of hyperalertness and reduces the need for sleep, leading to insomnia. The parasympathetic nerves (i.e., the visceral nerves that are part of the autonomic nervous system controlling heart rate, respiration, digestion, sexual arousal, and other systems) maintain a state of homeostasis when the body is not under stress. When activated by stress, the associated symptoms often have the opposite effect of what is seen when the sympathetic nervous system is in control. Cardiovascular responses can include decreased blood pressure and heart rate, feelings of faintness, or actual fainting. There can also be an increased need to urinate along with feelings of abdominal pain, nausea, and diarrhea. People may complain of feeling drowsy or the need for more sleep.

Sleep Needs for Older Adults

Older adults often take longer to fall asleep, awaken more frequently, and sleep less at night and more in the daytime than younger adults. About half of older adults have insomnia and about 65%–70% have combined sleeping disorders. External factors, such as health changes, social changes, and medications, can affect sleeping. Typically, slow-wave sleep begins to decrease in adolescence, and continues throughout life. By middle age, many people complain that they sleep less deeply and arouse more easily, especially in the second half of the night. Sleep may become fragmented with numerous transient arousal periods. By very old age, some people no longer experience stage 3 non-REM sleep although REM sleep remains at 20%–25%; however, people with Alzheimer's disease show decreased REM sleep. Some older adults experience phase advance and an increased need for sleeping time and napping, possibly because sleep is less efficient with frequent arousals.

Gender Differences

Gender differences in sleep have been studied, but studies have provided varying information. Research done by the Sleep Heart Health Study (1997) suggests that women sleep more effectively than men, beginning in adolescence and continuing through adulthood. As they age, men experience more deterioration of sleep than women:

- Increased stage 1 non-REM sleep
- Increased stage 2 non-REM sleep
- Higher apnea index
- Decreased slow-wave sleep
- Decreased REM sleep

Women tend to report more insomnia than men, but polysomnography does not support this, suggesting that underlying disorders or sleep state misperception may cause women to report insomnia more frequently. The incidence of obstructive sleep apnea syndrome in men is double that of women, especially with premenopausal women, but rates become more equal after women reach menopause. On the other hand, restless legs syndrome is more common in women (67%).

Menstrual Cycle

The menstrual cycle can affect sleep. The reproductive cycle includes:

Phase	Description	Effect
Follicular	The endometrial lining sheds (menstruation), and hormone levels of estradiol, progesterone, and LH decrease; FSH increases to develop a new follicle and renew the endometri-al lining. By the 4th day, estradiol levels rise, causing FSH levels to fall and LH levels to increase again.	OSAS increases: Upper airway swelling. Pain from abdominal cramping or profuse drain-age, which may impair sleep.
Ovulation	The dominant follicle secretes increased estradiol, causing the pituitary gland to secrete LH with a surge at days 11–13, causing follicular rupture and ovulation.	Discomfort during ovulation may impair sleep.
Luteal phase	Estradiol levels fall while progesterone levels increase 24 hours after ovulation, forming the corpus luteum from the ruptured follicle. The uterine lining enlarges. Without fertilization, both estradiol and progesterone levels fall, leading again to menstruation.	OSAS decreases: ↑Respiratory drive. ↑ Pharyngeal stability. ↑ Response to hypercapnia and hypoxia.

Abbreviations: LH = luteinizing hormone; FSH = follicle-stimulating hormone; and OSAS = obstructive sleep apnea syndrome.

Polycystic Ovarian Syndrome

Polycystic ovarian syndrome (PCOS) is an endocrine abnormality resulting in irregular menstrual cycles with rare or no ovulation and oligomenorrhea or amenorrhea, evidence of hyperandrogenism (virilization), and polycystic ovaries (found on ultrasound). Obesity is a common finding in PCOS as are acne, male pattern baldness, and hirsutism, resulting from increased testosterone production. The obesity combined with insulin resistance results in central obesity with enlargement of the abdomen and hyperinsulinism, which causes further increase in the production of male hormones (androgens). The obesity associated with PCOS markedly increases the risk for OSAS by 30–40 times over those at the same weight but without PCOS. Additionally, stress associated with changes in the body, such as alopecia and increased facial hair, may impair sleeping.

Metabolic Syndrome

Metabolic syndrome is a group of abnormalities, including the following:

- Abdominal obesity: Males, waist over 40 inches; females, waist over 35 inches
- Hypertension: 130/85 mm Hg or more
- High cholesterol levels (increased triglycerides and LDL and reduced HDL) and atherosclerosis
- Insulin resistance
- Fasting blood glucose 100 mg/dL or more
- Increased risk of blood clots and vascular inflammation.

In general, people who sleep less than 6 hours a night or 9–10 hours a night are at increased risk of weight gain and increased risk of metabolic syndrome. Patients often present with disrupted sleep patterns that coincide with increased weight and evidence of metabolic syndrome. Metabolic syndrome is associated with obstructive sleep apnea syndrome because of the impact obesity has on respiration.

Pregnancy

Pregnancy can affect the ability to sleep.

Trimester	Effects
First	Total sleep time (TST) increases about 30 minutes, and daytime sleepiness is common. Slow-wave sleep (SWS) declines. Progesterone levels rise, resulting in a hypnotic effect and increased respira-tory drive. Morning sickness may impair sleep in the morning.
Second	TST decreases to prepregnancy levels, and SWS returns to normal. Morning sickness usually declines. The hypnotic effect of progesterone declines but causes increased urination, which can impair sleep. As the fetus grows, the functional residual capacity reduces, respiration requires increased energy, and shortness of breath increases, disrupting sleep.
Third	TST remains at prepregnancy levels (although it may be slightly increased with daytime napping), but SWS and REM sleep decrease. Mechanical pressure from the growing fetus can impair breathing. Nocturia, leg cramps, back pain, acid reflux, and general discomfort may increase and interrupt sleep. Restless legs syndrome and periodic limb movement syndrome increase during pregnancy, further disrupting sleep.

Maternal Sleep

Maternal sleep may be markedly impaired, especially in the first few months after delivery when the mother must awaken every 2–3 hours to feed her infant. Total sleep time of 7 hours or less is common. Newborn infants usually nurse 8–12 times daily for 20–30 minutes each time, so mothers who are unable to nap in the daytime because of the need to care for other children or because of employment may suffer from sleep deprivation. Infants usually begin to establish a longer and more normal pattern of sleeping by 3 months of age, at which time the mother's sleeping pattern also returns to normal. Nursing mothers produce high levels of prolactin, which increases slow-wave sleep to about 43% (compared to 15% for mothers who bottle feed), so mothers who breastfeed may have more deep sleep. Bed sharing with the infant does not seem to have more of an impact on the mother's sleep than when the infant sleeps separately.

Menopause

Menopause occurs when amenorrhea persists for 12 months after the last menstruation. Hormonal changes can cause hot flashes, which are more common in the evening and at night, interrupting sleep and resulting in complaints of insomnia. Rates of obstructive sleep apnea syndrome increase markedly after menopause as fat distribution changes with increased fat about the waist and abdomen, and weight tends to increase. Nocturia and urinary urgency become more common and increasingly interrupt sleep. Some women report symptoms of depression, which can also impair sleep. Depression may result directly from hormonal changes or from anxiety about aging and bodily changes. While hormone replacement therapy (HRT) can relieve some of the symptoms that interfere with sleep, concerns about damage to the cardiovascular system have sharply curtailed prescriptions for HRT. "Male menopause" is an age-related reduction in testosterone and tends to be less abrupt because hormone levels decrease more slowly; however, low testosterone levels can result in insomnia or other disturbances of sleep.

Hypothyroidism and Hyperthyroidism

Hypothyroidism occurs when the thyroid produces inadequate levels of thyroid hormones. Patients may complain of excessive daytime sleepiness and general fatigue. Weight gain can contribute to obesity and result in obstructive sleep apnea. Hypothyroidism is characterized on polysomnography by decreased REM and stage 3 non-REM sleep, but these findings return to normal with hormone treatment. Myxedema, which can occur after prolonged severe hypothyroidism, may be characterized by changes in respiration with hypoventilation and carbon dioxide retention, resulting in coma.

Hyperthyroidism (thyrotoxicosis) usually results from excess production of thyroid hormones (Graves' disease) from immunoglobulins providing abnormal stimulation of the thyroid gland. Patients may experience hyperexcitability, poor heat tolerance, and diaphoresis (night sweats), pruritus, tachycardia, atrial fibrillation, and restless legs syndrome, all of which can interfere with sleep. Patients may complain of anxiety and exhaustion.

Fibromyalgia and Chronic Fatigue Syndrome

Fibromyalgia is a complex syndrome of disorders that include fatigue, chronic generalized muscle pain, and focal areas of tenderness, persisting for at least 3 months. The cause of fibromyalgia is not clear and has only recently been recognized as a distinct disorder. About 80% of patients with fibromyalgia also have episodes of central sleep apnea, which causes the person to arouse. Additionally, 40% or more people have restless legs syndrome or periodic limb movement disorder. Bruxism (grinding of the teeth) is also common. A polysomnogram typically shows that patients are able to go to sleep, but during deep non-REM sleep, alpha spiking occurs, resulting in feelings of chronic fatigue.

Chronic fatigue syndrome (CFS), a condition in which the patient complains of unrelenting fatigue, unrelated to activity, is also characterized by an alpha electroencephalogram sleep anomaly. Both fibromyalgia and CFS are characterized by increased sleep latency, decreased slow-wave sleep, reduced REM sleep, decreased sleep efficiency, and increased motor activity.

Schizophrenia

Schizophrenia is a psychotic disorder characterized by personality disintegration and distortion in the perception of reality, thought processes, and social development. Symptoms may include delusions, withdrawal, hallucinations, disorganized speech, catatonia, alogia (i.e., an inability to speak because of mental deficiency, mental confusion, or aphasia), avolition, and magical thinking. Additionally, patients may experience bizarre delusions, such as thought broadcasting and hearing voices. Patients may complain of sleep disruption, especially during psychotic episodes, and may have chronic difficulty falling asleep and staying asleep and frequent nightmares. Polysomnography shows reduction in stage 3 non-REM sleep and delta waves. The greater the reduction of delta activity, the more severe the symptoms. Both sleep onset latency and wake after sleep onset are increased; total sleep time is decreased by about 1 hour; sleep efficiency is reduced; and delta-wave counts are decreased in each minute of non-REM sleep as well as total delta-wave counts. REM latency may also be decreased. Long-term, changes occur in REM but not in short-wave sleep.

Bipolar Disorder

Bipolar disorder is characterized by manic episodes alternating with depressive episodes, occurring in varying patterns interspersed with periods of normal mood (euthymia). A manic episode is a distinct period characterized by extremely elevated mood, energy, and unusual thought patterns, causing impairment in occupational functioning and social activities for at least 1 week. Symptoms include grandiose beliefs, rapid speech, racing thoughts, reckless behavior, increased energy, a decreased need for sleep, and a lack of awareness of sleep deprivation. Polysomnography shows a decrease in total sleep time with the patient frequently awake during the latter part of the night, short REM latency, and an increased density of REM. The symptoms of the depressive phase of bipolar disorder are the opposite of the manic phase. Depressive episodes include feelings of hopelessness, self-loathing, and suicidal ideation. Patients may experience physical and mental sluggishness and report hypersomnia (not supported by a multiple sleep latency test).

PTSD

Post-traumatic stress disorder (PTSD) is an anxiety disorder that develops as a response to a severe emotional or physical trauma. The patient is typically numb at first but later has symptoms that may include excessive irritability, nightmares, flashbacks to the traumatic scene, and overreactions to sudden noises. Symptoms common to these traumatic experiences include the following:

- Overpowering terror, helplessness, and fear of being killed
- Recurrent intrusive thoughts of trauma in dreams (in both REM and non-REM sleep), during awake periods, or through persistent flashbacks; some people develop a sleep phobia because of fear of nightmares.
- Avoidance of thoughts or recollections about the trauma
- Avoidance of persons or situations that provoke the memory of the original trauma
- Diminished interest in activities or persons
- Increased startle reflex, sleep disturbances, outbursts of temper, and difficulty concentrating

PTSD is also associated with high rates of obstructive sleep apnea syndrome.

GAD

Generalized anxiety disorder (GAD) is an unrealistic apprehension and worry that persists for 6 or more months. Unlike phobias, this is a general anxiety that is not triggered by a specific object or situation. GAD may be accompanied by tension, sweating, irritability, and hypervigilance. It occurs more frequently in women than men and is common in the elderly. Up to 70% of affected people report difficulty sleeping, including insomnia and sleep deprivation, which may be related to symptoms, such as tremulousness and muscle tension, autonomic arousal (i.e., shortness of breath, tachycardia, dry mouth, diarrhea), depression, and generalized fear and anxiety. Polysomnography shows a delay in onset of sleep, decreased slow-wave sleep and total sleep time, increased stage 1 non-REM sleep, and frequent arousals during the first half of the night. The REM latency period is about 90 minutes long, within normal range, but REM density is decreased.

Phobias

Phobias are uncontrollable, unfounded, and persistent fears of specific objects, situations, or activities that actually pose no threat. If confronted with the item causing the fear, anxiety, sweating, and tachycardia may develop. In severe situations, a panic attack may develop. Phobias may be specific (e.g., animals, blood, situational) or social. Social phobias are characterized by fear of social or performance activities, resulting in anxiety or panic attacks, which the person recognizes as excessive but causes the person to avoid triggering situations. Onset is usually during adolescence and often occurs in those with a history of shyness. Phobias usually do not affect sleep unless the phobia is sleep-related. In that case, patients may be afraid to fall asleep. Fear of the dark usually does not impair sleeping unless the person is prevented from having a light on. In the case of social phobias, anticipatory fear before an event may interfere with sleep.

Panic Disorder

Panic disorder is characterized by chronic, repeated, and unexpected panic attacks, which present as overwhelming fear, apprehension, and terror when there is no specific cause. Panic attacks may last from minutes to several hours. Initial attacks usually occur in an anxiety-provoking situation, while successive attacks are spontaneous. Patients often report to an emergency department with shortness of breath and chest pain, believing they are having a heart attack or severe respiratory problems. Patients typically complain of multiple sleep problems, including difficulty falling and staying asleep and decreased total sleep time (TST) as panic attacks can occur during sleep, especially when associated with sleep deprivation. The panic attacks are not related to nightmares or night terrors, and patients do not show confusion or amnesia after awakening. Polysomnography during panic attacks show they develop during late stage 2 non-REM sleep or early stage 3 non-REM sleep. While slow-wave sleep is normal in patients with panic disorder, muscle activity increases. REM latency remains normal or increased with normal REM density. Sleep onset is delayed; TST is decreased; and sleep is less efficient.

OCD

Obsessive-compulsive disorder (OCD) is a disorder in which patients are plagued by obsessions or compulsions that interfere with employment and social, interpersonal, and other daily activities and last more than 1 hour daily.

- Obsessions are unwanted, repeated, and uncontrollable ideas, images, or urges that come to mind involuntarily despite attempts to ignore or suppress them.
- Compulsions are repeated, unwanted patterns of behavior (impulses) to perform apparently irrational or useless acts (e.g., washing hands, arranging and rearranging items) that are often responses to obsessions and done to reduce stress.

A sense of dread may develop if the compulsion is resisted, and some try to ignore or suppress thoughts or behaviors. Patients often have pronounced sleep disturbances because of their obsessions and compulsions, and their need to carry out repetitive behavior may make sleep studies difficult. They may resist any reusable equipment (e.g., masks) because of fear of germs. Polysomnography may show decreases in total sleep time, increased awakening, and decreased stage 3 non-REM sleep.

Major Depressive Disorder

Major depressive disorder is a depressed mood, profound and constant sense of hopelessness and despair, or loss of interest in all or almost all activities for a period of 2 weeks or more. Major depression varies in intensity and is characterized by a combination of symptoms that interfere with the ability to work, sleep, eat, and engage in activities. Symptoms include depressed mood, lack of interest, weight change, pessimism, and suicidal ideation. Complaints range from insomnia (a first symptom in about 40% and in 56% of relapses) to hypersomnia with constant daytime fatigue. Interestingly, sleep deprivation tends to reduce anxiety in depressed patients. Polysomnography shows increased sleep onset latency with periods of wakefulness, increased stage 1 non-REM sleep, and decreased slow-wave sleep, especially in the first non-REM sleep period. The REM latency period shortens to 30–50 minutes, and REM density increases. Antidepressants increase the REM latency period, decrease REM density, and decrease the overall percentage of REM sleep, especially during the first third of the sleep period.

Pulmonary Changes Associated with Aging

Pulmonary changes associated with aging typically include decreased pulmonary elasticity, decreases in alveolar surface area and size of airways, weakening of muscles of respiration (diaphragm and intercostals), and chest wall rigidity, so exchange of oxygen is impaired. Forced expiratory volume and forced vital capacity are also reduced. Overall strength is often decreased, so there is less ability to breathe deeply, and cough reflex and ciliary action are also decreased. Older adults may have less sensitivity to changes in oxygen and carbon dioxide levels (hypoxia, hypercapnia), so the increase in respiratory rate to compensate may be impaired and less noticeable. These changes may affect sleep in the older adult and may cause further decreases in oxygen saturation during episodes of sleep apnea. Episodes of hypoxia may be prolonged because of increased airway resistance.

COPD

Chronic obstructive pulmonary disease (COPD) causes limitations in airflow and may include both emphysema and chronic bronchitis, or more often a combination. The primary components of COPD include the following:

- Progressive airflow limitation
- Inflammatory response that causes a narrowing of the peripheral airways and thickening of the vessel walls of the pulmonary vasculature
- Exertional dyspnea and chronic cough

Acute exacerbation can result in decompensation with increased hypoxemia with oxygen saturation less than 90% with tachycardia, tachypnea, cyanosis, change in mental status, and hypercapnia. Dyspnea and orthopnea are common symptoms, so patients undergoing polysomnography may not be able to recline fully during testing. If COPD is severe, patients may sleep sitting upright in a chair. COPD when combined with sleep apnea–hypopnea can result in increased total sleep time, decreased sleeping efficiency, and a slight decrease in stage 1 non-REM sleep.

Pulmonary Hypertension

Pulmonary hypertension or pulmonary arterial hypertension (PAH) is a progressive disease that causes hypertension of the pulmonary arteries, restricting blood flow through the lungs and causing persistent hypoxia, especially on exertion. Primary PAH may result from immune responses, pulmonary emboli, sickle cell disease, collagen diseases, Raynaud's disease, and the use of contraceptives. Secondary PAH may result from pulmonary vasoconstriction caused by hypoxemia related to chronic obstructive pulmonary disease, sleep-disordered breathing, kyphoscoliosis, obesity, smoke inhalation, altitude sickness, interstitial pneumonia, and neuromuscular disorders. While PAH may be one direct cause of sleep-disordered breathing, all patients with PAH are at increased risk of sleep-disordered breathing and oxygen desaturation during sleep because of decreased ventilatory reserve; thus, oximetry should be carefully monitored as rates may fall to less than 90%, sometimes for prolonged periods of time.

Cardiovascular Changes Associated with Aging

Cardiovascular changes associated with aging may include existing heart disease, such as congestive heart failure, coronary artery disease, dysrhythmias, or hypertension that predispose them to a decrease in arterial elasticity with increased systolic blood pressure, widened pulse pressure, and larger pulse waves. Both resting and maximal heart rates may be reduced, making it more difficult for the body to respond to conditions that require increased oxygen, such as hypovolemia, hypotension, and hypoxia. Changes in the musculature of the left ventricle may result in decreased overall stroke volume. The changes with aging may also result in an increased incidence of hypertension or angina in response to sleep-disordered breathing. Dysrhythmias, such as atrial fibrillation, are more common in older adults and may be noted on polysomnogram.

Heart Failure

Heart failure (formerly known as congestive heart failure) is a cardiac disease that includes disorders of contractions (systolic dysfunction), filling (diastolic dysfunction), or both and may include pulmonary, peripheral, or systemic edema. The most common causes are coronary artery disease, systemic or pulmonary hypertension, cardiomyopathy, and valvular disorders. The incidence of chronic heart failure correlates with age. Heart failure may cause pulmonary edema that impairs ventilation, leading to hypoxia, especially when the patient is lying in supine position, such as during sleep. The circulatory time decreases overall, so changes in oximetry to show hypoxia may be delayed. The autonomic nervous system's regulation of breathing to control oxygen levels may be impaired, resulting in periodic breathing patterns, Cheyne-Stokes breathing, or central sleep apnea (CSA). Low rates of arterial carbon dioxide also correlate with CSA and Cheyne-Stokes breathing. Heart failure increases the risk of sleep apnea, predominately CSA, sleep disordered breathing, and insomnia. Patients with pulmonary edema may not be able to recline fully in the supine position for polysomnography.

Coronary Artery Disease

Coronary artery disease results in narrowing of the lumen of the coronary arteries, leading to ischemia of the cardiac muscle and angina pectoris, pain that may occur in the sternum, chest, neck, arms (especially the left), or back. The pain frequently occurs with crushing pain substernally, radiating down the left arm or both arms, although this type of pain is more common in men than women, whose symptoms may appear less acute and include nausea, shortness of breath, and fatigue. Elderly or diabetic patients may also have pain in the arms, no pain at all (silent ischemia), or weakness and numbness in arms. Stable angina episodes usually last for less than 5 minutes and are fairly predictable exercise-induced episodes caused by atherosclerotic lesions blocking 75% or more of the lumen of the effected coronary artery. Precipitating events include exercise, decrease in environmental temperature, heavy eating, strong emotions (e.g., fright, anger), or exertion, including coitus. Stable angina episodes usually resolve in less than 5 minutes by decreasing activity levels and administering sublingual nitroglycerine.

Unstable angina (also known as preinfarction or crescendo angina) is a progression of coronary artery disease and occurs when there is a change in the pattern of stable angina. The pain may increase, may not respond to a single nitroglycerine, and may persist for 5 minutes or more. Usually pain is more frequent, lasts longer, and may occur at rest. Unstable angina may indicate rupture of an atherosclerotic plaque and the beginning of thrombus formation so it should always be treated as a medical emergency as it may indicate a myocardial infarction.

Variant angina (also known as Prinzmetal's angina) results from spasms of the coronary arteries, either with or without atherosclerotic plaques, and is often related to smoking, alcohol, or illicit stimulants. Elevation of ST segments usually occurs with variant angina. Variant angina frequently occurs cyclically at the same time each day and often while the person is at rest, so it may occur during polysomnography.

Review Video: Coronary Artery Disease
Visit mometrix.com/academy and enter code: 950720

Dementia with Lewy Bodies

Dementia with Lewy bodies is characterized by cognitive and physical decline similar to Alzheimer's, but symptoms may fluctuate frequently. This form of dementia may include visual hallucinations, muscle rigidity, and tremors. Polysomnography is used for diagnosis because a primary characteristic is REM behavior disorder (RBD), a parasomnia in which the paralysis (atonia) that usually accompanies REM sleep is not present, so the person acts out activities of the dream, moving arms and sometimes grunting or shouting. RBD may also include sleepwalking and periodic leg movements. RBD is frequently one of the earliest symptoms, appearing before other indications of dementia. Polysomnography montage includes full electroencephalogram to rule out seizure disorders, video monitoring, and electromyogram for all extremities to monitor movement. A polysomnogram may be done to monitor the effectiveness of treatment with clonazepam. Patients with dementia may become increasingly confused and sometimes belligerent or combative, so the technologist should avoid arguing and should try to keep explanations and stimulation to a minimum.

Parkinson's Disease

Parkinson's disease is an extrapyramidal movement motor system disorder caused by loss of brain cells that produce dopamine. Typical symptoms include tremor of face and extremities, rigidity, bradykinesia, akinesia, poor posture, and lack of balance and coordination, causing increasing problems with mobility, talking, and swallowing. Some patients may suffer depression, mood changes, and dementia (about 30%). Tremors usually present unilaterally in an upper extremity. Disorders in sleep, including REM behavior disorder (RBD), may be an early symptom. Levodopa and Sinemet, commonly used to treat Parkinson's disease, may cause increased anxiety, insomnia, and nightmares. Monoamine oxidase inhibitors, such as Selegiline, are stimulants and may cause insomnia. Dopamine agonists, such as Requip, may cause increased drowsiness and sleep attacks. Sleep disorders associated with Parkinson's disease include obstructive sleep apnea, central sleep apnea, periodic breathing, and Cheyne-Stokes breathing. Restless legs syndrome is also common. During polysomnography, the patient may exhibit REM behavior disorder, frequently dislodging electrodes and other equipment, such as masks. Precautions to prevent falls should be observed.

Generalized Tonic–Clonic Seizures

Generalized tonic–clonic seizures are sudden involuntary abnormal electrical disturbances in the brain that can manifest as alterations of consciousness, spastic tonic, clonic movements, convulsions, and loss of consciousness. Seizures may be partial, affecting part of the brain, or generalized, affecting the whole brain. Seizures are characterized as focal (localized), focal with rapid generalization (spreading), and generalized (widespread). Some occur only during sleep or only during waking, but some may occur in either state. Interictal epileptiform activity (IEA) is epileptic-like electroencephalogram changes that commonly occur between seizures and during sleep.

Type/Sleep Association	Seizure Activity
Generalized tonic–clonic: Seizures occur in non-REM sleep. IEA increases during non-REM sleep (especially at sleep onset) and then decreases in REM sleep.	Tonic period (10–30 seconds): eyes roll upward with loss of consciousness, arms flex, body stiffens in symmetric tonic contraction, apneic with cyanosis and salivating
	Clonic period (10 seconds to 30 minutes, but usually 30 seconds): violent rhythmic jerking with contraction and relaxation; may be incontinent of urine and feces; contractions slow and then stop

Primary Generalized Myoclonus Epilepsy

Primary generalized myoclonus epilepsy is related to the epileptiform discharges during sleep.

Types	Seizure Activity/Sleep Association
Primary generalized myoclonus	Brief jerking motions, most common upon awakening: Primary generalized myoclonic seizures occur during both spontaneous and induced arousals. Both myoclonus and interictal epileptic-form activity (IEA) with polyspike and polyspike-wave discharges may occur.
Absence (petit mal)	Onset is between 4–12 years of age and usually ends in puberty. Onset is abrupt with brief loss of consciousness for 5–10 seconds and slight loss of muscle tone, but the patient often appears to be daydreaming. It may include lip smacking or eye twitching. Characterized on electroencephalogram by 3-Hz spike-wave complexes. IEA activation varies during non-REM sleep. Sleep stage 1 non-REM: Bursts shorten but with well-defined spikes. Sleep stage 2 non-REM: There are irregular bursts with polyspikes; independent focal spikes occur in right and left frontal areas. Sleep stage 3 non-REM: There is a decline in rhythm of spiking and a decrease in the rate of repetitions to 0.5–2 Hz. REM sleep: This is similar to the wake state with generalized discharges, but they are of short duration.

Generalized Epilepsy

The type of generalized epilepsy, such as Lennox-Gastaut and West syndromes, is related to the epileptiform discharges during sleep.

Types	Seizure Activity/Sleep Association
Lennox-Gastaut syndrome	This is a severe intractable seizure disorder with multiple types of seizures, occurring throughout waking and sleeping, and intellectual disabilities. Tonic-clonic seizures are common on awakening and may occur during sleep. Tonic seizures are most common during sleep: Generalized, slow, spike-wave complexes of 2.5 Hz or more; Increase in activity during non-REM sleep with polyspikes and bursts of rapid activity at 10–20 Hz; Prolonged or continuous spike-wave discharges (usually inversely correlated to the degree of intellectual disabilities)
West syndrome	This is characterized by brain damage, resulting in infantile spasms, intellectual disabilities, and interictal electroencephalogram (EEG) hypsarrhythmia (multi-focal and generalized high-voltage spikes with disorganized background tracing). Seizures usually occur while awake, although EEG abnormalities are evident during sleep: Increase in interictal epileptiform activity with spikes and slow-wave discharges, occurring periodically during non-REM sleep; Decrease in hypsar-rhythmia (irregular spikes), occurring during REM sleep

Focal or Partial Seizures

Focal or partial seizures are caused by an electrical discharge to a localized area of the cerebral cortex, such as the frontal, temporal, or parietal lobes, with seizure characteristics related to the area of involvement. They may begin in a focal area and become generalized, often preceded by an aura.

- Simple partial: Unilateral motor symptoms including somatosensory, psychic, and autonomic
  - Aversive: Eyes and head turned away from focal side
  - Sylvan (usually during sleep): Tonic–clonic movements of the face, salivation, and arrested speech
- Special sensory: Various sensations (e.g., numbness, tingling, prickling, pain) spreading from one area; may include visual sensations, posturing, or hypertonia; rare in patients younger than 8 years of age
- Complex (psychomotor): No loss of consciousness but altered consciousness and nonresponsive with amnesia; may involve complex sensorium with bad tastes, auditory or visual hallucinations, déjà vu, or strong fear; may carry out repetitive activities, such as walking, running, smacking lips, chewing, or drawling; rarely aggressive; seizure usually followed by prolonged drowsiness and confusion; occurs throughout adolescence

Frontal Lobe Epilepsy and Temporal Lobe Epilepsy

Frontal lobe epilepsy and temporal lobe epilepsy are related to epileptiform discharges and seizure activity during sleep.

Subtypes	Seizure Activity/Sleep Association
Benign focal epilepsy of childhood (Rolandic epilepsy)	Seizures are either generalized tonic–clonic or unilateral focal motor with oropharyngeal sensorimotor phenomena (e.g., hypersalivation, guttural sounds). Most seizures (75%) are nocturnal and are not associated with cognitive impairment. Interictal epileptiform activity (IEA) is especially evident during stage 3 non-REM sleep with interictal spikes.
Supplementary sensorimotor	Seizures usually occur during sleep and are characterized by tonic posturing of extremities, usually asymmetrically with upper extremities. Electroencephalogram (EEG) shows interictal, high-amplitude, transient or sharp waves, maximum at vertex, with an electrodecremental pattern.
Nocturnal frontal	Seizures vary widely and include brief (< 20 seconds) paroxysmal arousal that may include sitting upright and vocalizing, nocturnal paroxysmal dystonia (20–120 seconds) with dystonic posturing and vocalizations, or episodic nocturnal wandering (1–3 minutes). Surface EEGs may not indicate activity during seizures, but IEA are evident with flattening of background, rhythmic theta and delta activity, and sharp waves (frontal).

Temporal Lobe Epilepsy and Electrical Status Epilepticus of Sleep

Temporal lobe epilepsy and electrical status epilepticus of sleep (ESES) are related to epileptiform activity.

Temporal lobe epilepsy	Seizure activity is less frequent during sleep, although it does occur in some patients.
	Increase in interictal epileptiform activity (IEA) in non-REM sleep with high-frequency spikes and contralateral focal discharges
	Decrease in REM sleep

ESES	ESES is typically nonconvulsive but involves extensive epileptiform activity during sleep and cognitive impairment. It may be associated with Landau-Kleffner syndrome and loss of language skills. Characteristics of ESES include the following: Continuous spiking during slow-wave sleep, stage 3 non-REM with spike-wave complexes at 2–2.5 Hz Reduction in pattern during REM sleep and wake state
Landau-Kleffner syndrome	This disorder, also known as infantile acquired aphasia, involves sudden or gradual onset of loss of language skills and is characterized by nocturnal multifocal spikes and spike-wave discharges, although seizures are rare.
	IEA in 85% or more of slow-wave sleep

Amyotrophic Lateral Sclerosis

Amyotrophic lateral sclerosis (ALS) is a degenerative disease of the motor neurons from the anterior horns of the spinal cord and the motor nuclei in the lower brainstem. The neurons begin to die, and the muscles to which they are attached atrophy and weaken. Symptoms include increasing muscle weakness, twitching, spasticity, fatigue, and lack of coordination. Weakness of facial and pharyngeal muscles impairs the ability to swallow and cough, increasing the risk of aspiration and obstructive sleep apnea. As respiratory muscles weaken, patients often develop central alveolar hypoventilation, requiring mechanical ventilation. Because of generalized weakness, patients may have difficulty following instructions required for physiological calibrations. Additionally, patients may need assistance to move or turn during the night and may need the head of the bed elevated. If patients have difficulty exhaling, then bi-level-positive airway pressure is usually preferred over continuous positive airway pressure.

Centers for Disease Control Isolation Guidelines

The Centers for Disease Control isolation guidelines include both standard precautions that apply to all patients and transmission-based precautions for those with known or suspected infections. Standard precautions should be used during poly-somnography for all patients because all body fluids (i.e., sweat, urine, feces, blood, sputum), nonintact skin, and mucous membranes may be infected.

Hand hygiene	Wash hands before and after each patient contact.
Personal Protective equipment (PPE)	Use PPE, such as gloves, gowns, and masks, eye protection, or face shields, depending on the patient's condition and degree of exposure.
Respiratory hygiene/ cough etiquette	Educate staff, patients, family, and visitors, and post instructions that are language appropriate. Use source control measures, such as covering cough, disposing of tissues, using surgical mask on person coughing or on staff to prevent inhalation of droplets, and properly dispose of dressings and used equipment. Wash hands after contact with respiratory secretions, and maintain a distance of 3 feet or more from coughing person when possible.
Safe injection practice	Use sterile single-use needles and syringes one time only, and discard safely.

Transmission-based precautions apply to those patients known or suspected infections as well as those with excessive wound drainage, other discharge, or fecal incontinence. Transmission-based precautions include the following:

Contact	Use personal protective equipment, including gown and gloves, for all contacts with the patient or patient's immediate environment. Maintain patient in a private room or 3 feet or more away from other patients.
Droplet	Use a mask while caring for the patient (appropriate for influenza, *Streptococcus* infection, pertussis, rhinovirus, adenovirus, and pathogens that remain viable and infectious for only short distances).
	Maintain patient in a private room or 3 feet or more away from other patients with a curtain separating them. Use a mask for the patient if transporting the patient from one area to another.
Airborne	Place patient in an airborne infection isolation room (appropriate for measles, chickenpox, tuberculosis, and severe acute respiratory syndrome because pathogens remain viable and infectious for long distances). Use N95 respirators (or masks) while caring for the patient.

RACE Guidelines

In response to a fire, the sleep technologist must immediately take action to protect the patient and sound an alarm, and use the RACE guidelines.

Rescue	Remove patient from danger.
Alarm	Sound the alarm to alert others, including the fire department.
Contain	Use extinguishers as appropriate (using multipurpose initially if that is all that is available): Class A: For combustibles, such as wood and paper, use water. Class B: For flammable liquids, such as solvents, paints, gasoline, use dry chemical extinguishers. Class C: For electrical equipment, use carbon dioxide and dry-chemical extinguishers. Extinguishers for Class A and Class B fires can be used if the current is turned off. Class D: For combustible metals, such as magnesium, titanium, sodium, potassium, use special dry compound powders, such as powdered graphite, sodium chloride, talc, or dry sand.
Evacuate	Exit the area of the fire immediately, and evacuate the entire building if the fire is not completely contained in a very small area (e.g., a waste can) as fire can spread rapidly and unpredictably.

Medical Emergencies

Myocardial Infarction

Myocardial infarction (MI) occurs when there is an imbalance between the heart's demand for oxygen and the supply. An MI may occur after an episode of unstable angina caused by rupture of an atherosclerotic plaque and thrombosis associated with coronary artery spasm, but it may also result from vasoconstriction, acute blood loss, decreased oxygen, and cocaine ingestion. Symptoms of MI vary considerably, with men having the more "classic" symptom of sudden crushing chest pain and women and those under 55 presenting with atypical symptoms. Diabetic patients may have a reduced sensation of pain because of neuropathy, complaining primarily of weakness. Elderly patients may also have neuropathic changes that reduce the sensation of pain. Symptoms may include blood pressure changes, palpitations, angina, dyspnea, pulmonary or peripheral edema, pallor, cold clammy skin, and diaphoresis. Polysomnography may show changes in respiration, electrocardiographic changes (e.g., ST segment and T-wave changes), tachycardia, bradycardia, and dysrhythmias), and decreased oxygen saturation with hypoxia. Patient may need oxygen or cardiopulmonary resuscitation. Emergency assistance should be requested.

Acute Asthma Attack

An acute asthma attack is precipitated by some stimulus, such as an antigen that triggers an allergic response, resulting in an inflammatory cascade that causes edema of the mucous membranes (swollen airway), contraction of smooth muscles (bronchospasm), increased mucus production (cough and obstruction), and hyperinflation of airways (decreased ventilation and shunting). While asthma is more common in children, older adults are also affected but may be misdiagnosed. Older adults may complain of daytime sleepiness and increased asthma symptoms during the night, characterized by wheezing, dyspnea, and coughing. In cough-variant asthma, a severe cough may be the only symptom, at least initially. Bronchodilators should be available to relieve symptoms as patients may become hypoxic. With chronic asthma, permanent damage to airways may cause decreased oxygen saturation during sleep and disordered sleep. If nocturnal hypoxia is severe, the patient may require supplemental oxygen (1–2 L/min).

Stroke

Strokes (cerebrovascular accidents) result from interruption of the blood flow to an area of the brain. About 80% of strokes are ischemic, resulting from blockage of an artery supplying the brain because of thrombosis in a large artery, lacunar infarct (penetrating thrombosis in small artery), or embolism. Hemorrhagic strokes result from a ruptured cerebral artery, causing not only a lack of oxygen and nutrients but also edema that causes widespread pressure and damage. Strokes most commonly occur in the right or left hemisphere, but the exact location and the extent of brain damage affects the type of presenting symptoms. If the frontal area of either side is involved, there tends to be memory and learning deficits. Typical presenting symptoms include slurred speech or aphasia, loss of consciousness, weakness or paralysis on one side of the body, headache, and sudden onset of vision disturbances or confusion. A stroke is always a medical emergency that requires immediate intervention as some treatments, such as thrombolytics to dissolve clots, should be initiated within 3 hours.

Diabetic Ketoacidosis

Diabetic ketoacidosis (DKA) is a complication of diabetes mellitus. Inadequate production of insulin results in glucose being unavailable for metabolism, so lipolysis (i.e., breakdown of fat) produces free fatty acids as an alternate fuel source. Glycerol in both fat cells and the liver is converted to ketone bodies, which are used for cellular metabolism less efficiently than glucose. The ketone bodies lower serum pH, leading to ketoacidosis. Symptoms include:

- Kussmaul respirations, which is hyperventilation to eliminate a buildup of carbon dioxide, associated with "ketone breath"
- Fluid imbalance, including loss of potassium and other electrolytes, resulting in dehydration and diuresis with excess thirst
- Cardiac arrhythmias, related to potassium loss, leading to cardiac arrest
- Ketonuria
- Hyperglycemia (elevated glucose); normal values (fasting):
    - Neonate: 40–60 mg/dL
    - Younger than12 months: 50–90 mg/dL
    - Child: 60–100 mg/dL
    - Adult: 65–99 mg/dL or up to 125 mg/dL (diabetics)

Glucose testing should be done immediately if DKA is suspected and a physician notified as treatment with insulin must be initiated.

Acute Hypoglycemia

Acute hypoglycemia (hyperinsulinism) may result from pancreatic islet tumors, hyperplasia, increased insulin production, or the use of insulin to control diabetes mellitus. Hyperinsulinism can cause damage to the central nervous and cardiopulmonary systems, interfering with the functioning of the brain and causing neurological impairment. Too little food, too much insulin, or too much exercise can all trigger hypoglycemia in the diabetic. Symptoms include the following:

- Blood glucose less than 40 mg/dL in neonates and less than 50–60 mg/dL for others
- Central nervous system: seizures, altered consciousness, lethargy, and poor feeding with vomiting, myoclonus, respiratory distress, diaphoresis, hypothermia, and cyanosis
- Adrenergic system: diaphoresis, tremor, tachycardia, palpitation, hunger, and anxiety

Treatment depends on the underlying cause, but glucose/glucagon should be available during the polysomnogram for patients who take insulin and should be administered immediately with signs of hypoglycemia, supported by blood glucose testing. The physician should be notified as other medications may be indicated to increase blood glucose levels.

CPR

The American Heart Association guidelines for cardiopulmonary resuscitation (CPR) include the ABC method.

A	Airway	Tilt the head back to open the airway, supporting the back of the head and pulling the chin upward.
B	Breathing	Provide two 1-second breaths initially and then: Two rescuers: Use a compression to breathing rate of 30:2 for adults and 15:2 for children and infants. One rescuer: Use a compression to breathing rate of 30:2 for all ages.
C	Circulation	A compression rate of 100/min for all ages with two hands for adults, the heel of one hand for children, and two to three fingers for infants: Adults and children: Compress lower half of sternum, between nipples, to a depth of 1.5–2 inches. Infants: Compress lower half of sternum, immediately below nipple line, to a depth of one-third to one-half chest depth, depending on age.

Continue CPR until there is a return of a pulse, breathing, or defibrillation with an automated external defibrillator. If the heart remains beating, but respiratory arrest is present, do rescue breathing with two initial 1-second breaths followed by subsequent breaths every 5–6 seconds for adults and 3–5 seconds for children and infants.

Airway Obstruction

With airway obstruction, the person usually begins coughing. If the person can respond verbally to the question, "Are you choking?" the airway is not completely obstructed. The patient is encouraged to cough up the foreign body; however, if the person cannot respond, loses consciousness, or becomes cyanotic, intervention is needed.

- Adults/children (sitting or standing, conscious): Wrap arms around the torso from behind with the patient leaning slightly forward. Place one fist against the diaphragm (below the ribs) and lock in place with the other hand. Pull sharply inward and upward to force air out of the lungs. Repeat as necessary or until the patient becomes unconscious.
- Adults/children (unconscious or supine): Place the heel of one hand on the diaphragm, cover with other hand and compress inward and upward for five thrusts. Begin cardiopulmonary resuscitation (CPR) if there is no response.
- Infants: Hold the child in a prone position with the head and thorax angling downward and do five backslaps between shoulder blades. Follow with five abdominal thrusts. It this is not effective, begin CPR.

Treatment and Intervention

Narcolepsy Intervention

Narcolepsy intervention includes a number of measures to maintain wakefulness and prevent the person from falling asleep during waking hours.

- Stimulants:
  - Amphetamines (dextroamphetamine, Dexedrine; methamphetamine, Desoxyn), or amphetamine-like drugs (methylphenidate, Ritalin) decrease daytime sleepiness and reduce daytime sleeping but may cause hypertension, tachycardia, anxiety, headache, and gastrointestinal problems. The potential for abuse exists.
  - Modafinil (Provigil), a dopamine agonist, is similar in action to amphetamines but has fewer side effects so it is usually the preferred drug.
- Tricyclic antidepressants (TCAs): TCAs (protriptyline, clomipramine, desipramine) reduce REM sleep, control cataplexy, and reduce hypnagogic or hypnopompic hallucinations and sleep paralysis. Adverse effects include dry mouth, muscle twitching, constipation, tachycardia, urinary retention, confusion, appetite changes, hypotension, and sexual dysfunction.
- Selective serotonin re-uptake inhibitors (SSRIs) SSRI antidepressants (fluoxetine, paroxetine, sertraline, and venlafaxine) work similarly to TCAs but usually have fewer adverse effects. Adverse effects can include apathy, appetite changes, increased depression, suicidal ideation, tremors, bruxism (grinding teeth), and sexual dysfunction.

Obstructive Sleep Apnea Interventions

Conservative obstructive sleep apnea (OSA) interventions usually include continuous positive airway pressure although surgery may also be recommended as a last resort. However, intervention usually begins by eliminating those factors that may influence the condition. In mild cases, conservative intervention alone may be sufficient.

- Avoid drinking any alcohol in the evening as it may increase sleep apnea.
- Stop smoking as it impairs airways.
- Treat allergies, which may cause swelling and obstruction of airways.
- Control obesity by diet and exercise.
- Avoid night shift work, if possible.

- Review medications with the physician as some (e.g., tranquilizers, short-acting β-blockers) may increase apnea, especially if taken in the evening.
- Change sleep position if polysomnography indicates OSA occurs only in one position (e.g., while supine), although this alone is usually not sufficient treatment for most people as it can be difficult to control sleep positions even with bolsters and pillows.

POTENTIAL THERAPIES

Potential therapies for obstructive sleep apnea (OSA) include diet control. Obesity is one of the primary risk factors for OSA, especially for those with central obesity, affecting 40%–90% of OSA patients. Studies indicate that losing 10%–15% of weight can reduce OSA by 50% (as measured by the apnea–hypopnea index). Obesity can result in collapse of the upper airway and hypoventilation during sleep.

Diet/weight loss	Diet management includes a nutritional assessment and a diet plan, often low fat or low carbohydrate. Patients are usually encouraged to create a food diary to keep track of their meals. Most patients need ongoing support to stay on a diet. Support groups may benefit some patients.
Bariatric surgery	In some cases, bariatric surgery may be recommended if the patient is not able to lose weight and the obesity is severely compromising respirations/ventilation.

Potential therapies for obstructive sleep apnea (OSA) include the following:

Continuous positive airway pressure (CPAP)	Education regarding the CPAP devices should include the different types of masks and machines available.
	Bi-level positive airway pressure changes pressure during exhalation to facilitate breathing.
	Auto positive airway pressure has adjustable rather than fixed pressure.
	The technologist should explain the importance of using a humidifier to prevent the drying of mucous membranes, and the patient should understand that using CPAP is not a temporary or part-time solution but should be used with every sleep, whether at night or napping during the day.
Oral/dental devices	Some patients with mild OSA may be prescribed oral or dental devices, which fit inside the mouth or are fastened around the head to open the airway during sleep. Devices include the following: • Mandibular repositioning • Tongue retaining Patients should be cautioned to have devices fitted by professionals, such as a dentist, to avoid damage to the teeth, mouth, or jaw.

Potential therapies for obstructive sleep apnea include several recommended surgeries, especially for patients who resist using continuous positive airway pressure (CPAP) or for whom CPAP alone is ineffective. Surgical procedures include:

Tonsillectomy/ adenoidectomy (T&A)	Enlarged tonsils and adenoids may effectively block the airway, especially in children, so a T&A may prove curative. The T&A is often the treatment of choice rather than CPAP for children because CPAP may be ineffective if the tonsils and adenoids are markedly enlarged. However, children who are obese may still require CPAP after surgery.
Nasal reconstruction	If apnea is related to nasal obstruction from a deviated septum, overgrowth of tissue in the turbinates, or a narrowed nasal valve, then nasal reconstruction may alleviate this obstruction. In some cases, surgery is necessary to facilitate use of CPAP. Radiosurgical procedures may be used to remove excess tissue.

Potential therapies for obstructive sleep apnea (OSA) include a number of surgical procedures.

Uvulopalatopharyngo-plasty (UPPP)	If OSA relates to a narrowed airway, the excess tissue may be removed from the uvula and the soft palate, and the tonsils and adenoids are also removed. If the tongue is obstructive, tissue may be removed from the tongue as well (uvulopalatopharyngogloss-oplasty). Tongue reduction can also be done through radio-surgery. The UPPP is painful but is used for patients who do not or cannot use continuous positive airway pressure, and it may be an option rather than a tracheotomy for severe cases. Complications can include a feeling that a foreign body is in the throat and reflux of fluids/food through the nasal passages while swallowing.
Uvulopalatal flap (UPF)	The UPF removes minimal tissue from the soft palate, lifting it and removing the tonsils to increase the size of the airway. This is less invasive than the UPPP, but it still can be quite painful. It may be combined with other procedures, such as genioglossus advancement and radiosurgical tongue reduction.

Potential therapies for obstructive sleep apnea include a number of surgical procedures.

Genioglossus advancement (GA)	GA enlarges the hypopharyngeal area and is recommended for individuals whose tongues fall back and obstruct the airway. The genioglossus muscle attaches the tongue to the lower jaw at a bony prominence; GA moves this prominence forward and reattaches the tongue in a more anterior position, preventing the tongue from blocking the airway. This procedure may be done along with uvulopalatal flap and radiosurgical tongue reduction. GA is often more successful than uvulopalatopharyngoplasty
Hyoid myotomy (HM)	HM enlarges the hypopharyngeal area by pulling the hyoid bone forward, opening the airway; it is indicated for those with airway blockage at the epiglottis or base of the tongue. This procedure may be done in conjunction with GA or alone.

Potential therapies for obstructive sleep apnea (OSA) include a number of surgical procedures.

Maxillomandibular advancement (MMA)	MMA is recommended for patients with severe OSA that does not respond to other surgical treatments or continuous positive airway pressure, especially related to anatomic abnormalities (e.g., micrognathia) that narrow the airway. Both the mandible and maxilla are fractured on both sides; metal spacers are placed between the bones, and the midface is brought forward up to about 12 mm to enlarge the posterior airway. GA and nasal surgery may also be indicated. This procedure may change the appearance of the face.
Maxillomandibular expansion (MME)	MME is recommended for those whose jaws are not wide enough and involves cutting into both sides of the mandible and maxilla and placing distractors, which essentially stretch and expand the jaw, leaving a gap between the teeth, which is later corrected with orthodontia. This procedure may slightly change the appearance of the face.

Potential therapies for obstructive sleep apnea (OSA) include a number of surgical procedures.

Pillar procedure	The Pillar minimally invasive procedure is used to treat obstruction caused by the soft palate. It involves suturing three small inserts into the soft palate to provide support. This treatment is effective for mild-to-moderate OSA.
Tracheostomy	An opening directly into the trachea bypasses the obstruction and opens the airway, but it is invasive and can result in many complications, so it is now rarely done. When used to treat sleep disorders, the tracheostomy can be blocked during waking hours and opened during sleep. This procedure is primarily used as a last resort only in the elderly, the morbidly obese, those with facial abnormalities that preclude other treatments, and those with severe hypoxemia or cardiac arrhythmias.

Potential therapies for obstructive sleep apnea (OSA) include a number of surgical procedures.

Radiofrequency somnoplasty	This minimally invasive surgical technique uses low-power radiofrequency to create volumetric lesions in submucosal tissue. In a period lasting up to 8 weeks, the tissue is slowly absorbed, and the volume is decreased. The treatments are done under local anesthesia, and some swelling and mild discomfort may persist for 2–3 weeks: Nasal obstruction and snoring: Radiofrequency targets the nasal turbinates. Tongue: Multiple sessions at low-energy levels may be required to prevent swelling and irritation. Soft palate: Treatments strengthen and provide support to the soft palate.
Laser-assisted uvuloplasty (LAUP)	LAUP uses a laser to remove soft tissue of the uvula and soft palate to reduce snoring and open the airway. Surgery involves a series of laser treatments and may cause significant pain.

SAD

Seasonal affective disorder (SAD) is characterized by seasonal episodes of depression (usually fall and winter), increased appetite, and hypersomnia, requiring over 2.5 hours extra sleep a day during the fall and winter months. SAD may be related to chemical or hormonal changes in the brain because of reduced exposure to sunlight. Sleep is characterized by decreased efficiency, decreased delta sleep, and increased REM density with normal REM latency. Treatment includes the following:

Medications	Antidepressants
	Mood stabilizers (with bipolar disorder)
	Melatonin supplements
Phototherapy	Increased sun exposure. Light/phototherapy boxes (most common treatment): Treatments typically are given in the morning, beginning with 30-minute periods at 10,000 lux or 2-hour periods for 2500 lux boxes. The light box is placed 8–12 inches in front of the person while she or he eats, reads, or works at a computer.
	Dawn simulators: Low-intensity light is timed to turn on at about 5 am and gradually increases in brightness to mimic daybreak.

Bipolar patients with SAD who take mood stabilizers should be monitored carefully before light therapy because it may trigger manic episodes.

Circadian Rhythm Sleep Disorder

Circadian rhythm sleep disorders are characterized by advanced-phase sleep disorders, delayed-phase sleep disorders, free running, shift-work disorders, and other irregular patterns. Treatment includes the following:

Manipulating phase-response curve	To promote phase delay: Expose to light immediately before time of minimum body temperature (about 3 am). Avoid early morning light or wear sunglasses, and seek bright light in the evening.
	To promote phase advance: Expose to light after the time of minimum body temperature. Walk outside in sunlight after awakening and avoid bright light in the evening. Take melatonin supplements in the evening.
Accommodation	Adapt lifestyle to changes.
Chronotherapy	Monitor the phase delay or phase advance until a normal phase is reached, and then institute measures to prevent delay or advance.

RLS and PLMS

Restless legs syndrome (RLS) and periodic limb movements of sleep (PLMS) can both impair sleeping. The same treatments are used for both.

Dopamine agonists	Ropinirole (Requip) reduces the need to move the legs but may cause sudden episodes of sleeping, nausea, or constipation. Levodopa may also reduce symptoms but is associated with a wide range of adverse effects (e.g., orthostatic hypotension, insomnia, hallucinations). Pergolide is effective for both RLS and PLMS but can result in pleural fibrosis and valvular heart disease.
Non ergot agonist	Pramipexole has rapid onset for relief of RLS. Adverse effects are similar to those of ropinirole.

Benzodiazepines	Clonazepam depresses the central nervous system and allows the patient increased sleep but does not completely eradicate RLS or PLMS and may cause excess sedation and drug tolerance.
Opioids	Oxycodone and propoxyphene relieve symptoms for some people but have addictive qualities and may produce sedation and gastrointestinal upsets (e.g., constipation, nausea, vomiting).
Anticonvulsants	Gabapentin may relieve RLS but has many adverse effects, including sedation, fatigue, hypersomnolence, ataxia, and dizziness.

Insomnia and Cognitive-Behavioral Therapies

Insomnia can be difficult to treat because patients have developed habits of sleeping or have co-morbid conditions, such as personality or psychiatric disorders, which may interfere with treatment. Additionally, some patients may use alcohol or over-the-counter drugs to help them sleep, and some gain attention through their complaints.

Cognitive-behavioral therapies include the following:

Cognitive therapy	Using methods to stop worrying and obsessing about sleep to decrease arousal
Control of stimuli	Reducing behaviors that interfere with sleep
Phototherapy	Using bright lights to control circadian rhythm
Paradoxical intention	Telling the patient to stay awake (may be helpful for a select few patients)
Relaxation techniques	Practicing self-hypnosis and meditation
Sleep hygiene	Establishing habits that promote sleep
Sleep restriction	Going to bed and getting up at prescribed times (within 30 minutes of total sleep time that the patient reports or 5 hours); extending time slowly to maximum, if patient is able to sleep 85% of this time but not stay in bed beyond time actually sleeping (5 hours or more)

Sleep Hygiene

Sleep hygiene, that is, those methods, things, and activities that help patients to fall and stay asleep, must be understood by patients. While sleep hygiene is usually not sufficient to treat chronic insomnia, it may help those with milder insomnia or other sleep-related disorders. Methods include the following:

- Use the bed only for sleeping (or sex) but not for other activities, such as watching television or reading.
- Get out of bed after 20 minutes if not asleep and do something relaxing (e.g., reading) until sleepy.
- Do not sleep anywhere except in bed, and only go to bed when sleepy.
- Do something relaxing (e.g., reading, meditating) for 10–20 minutes before going to bed.
- Engage in activities that promote sleep, such as exercise in the afternoon or early evening, or a bedtime snack.
- Avoid activities that interfere with sleep, such as smoking, drinking caffeinated drinks, using alcohol, or taking daytime naps.

INSOMNIA MEDICATIONS

Insomnia can be treated effectively with medications as they offer fast relief of symptoms, but there are many adverse effects associated with drugs, including habituation, sedation, confusion, disorientation, and rebound insomnia when the drugs are withdrawn, so they are often combined with other treatments. Medications include antidepressants.

Tricyclics **Amitriptyline** **Doxepin** **Nortriptyline** **Trimipramine**	Increase total sleep time (TST), REM latency period, stage 1 and 2 non-REM sleep. Decrease REM sleep and sleep latency period.	Associated with numerous adverse effects: dry mouth, dry eyes, constipation, urinary retention, hypotension, tachycardia, confusion, and impaired memory; high risk of overdosage
Sedatives **Mirtazapine** **Nefazodone** **Trazodone**	Increase sleep continuity, TST, and REM latency period. Nefazodone only increases REM sleep and short-wave sleep.	Associated adverse effects: blurred vision, dry mouth, dry eyes, constipation, dizziness, lightheadedness, drowsiness, tremors, and incoordination

Medications for insomnia include the hypnotics, which are the most commonly used. They have similar effects on sleep, but adverse effects vary. These drugs have been associated with abnormal sleep behavior ("sleep driving") and allergic reactions. Hypnotics include the benzodiazepines.

General Effects	Drug Specific
Increased beta activity on electro-encephalogram and spindle activity Decreased sleep latency and wake time, following onset of sleep, slow-wave sleep, and REM sleep	Flurazepam: long half-life (especially in elderly patients) and rapid absorption with sedation, persisting into daytime hours, increasing confusion and disorientation and risk of injury Estazolam: intermediate half-life and rapid absorption; may be used with elderly patients Quazepam: long half-life and rapid absorption; should be avoided with elderly patients and those with pulmonary disorders Temazepam: intermediate half-life and slow absorption rate (peaking in 1–3 hours) but not associated with daytime sleepiness Triazolam: short half-life and rapid absorption, but not associated with daytime sleepiness, although may cause anxiety and amnesia

Insomnia medications, include nonbenzodiazepine hypnotics, which are commonly used for short-term treatment of insomnia. These medications usually target gamma-aminobutyric acid sites that control sleep, and most do not cause sedation or respiratory depression. Nonbenzodiazepine hypnotics include the following:

General Effects	Drug Specific
Increase total sleep time but do not affect REM sleep or short-wave sleep	Eszopiclone (Lunesta): This drug maintains sleep for 7–8 hours and can cause sleepiness in the daytime if people have to awaken early, and it can be habit-forming. Ramelteon (Rozerem): This medication does not target the central nervous system but rather the sleep–wake cycle and can be used long-term for those with difficulty with sleep onset. Adverse effects (rare) include dizziness, somnolence, and fatigue. Zaleplon (Ambien CR): The plain Ambien helped people fall asleep but did not maintain sleep well, but the CR version with extended release maintains sleep better for 7–8 hours. Zolpimist is a nasal spray with the same active ingredient. Zolpidem (Sonata): This medication is short acting, so it can be taken in the middle of the night if necessary without causing daytime sleepiness.

Signs of Violence and Aggression

Recognizing signs of violence or aggression is a skill needed by the sleep technologist who must intervene in a timely manner.

- Violence is a physical act perpetrated against an inanimate object, animal, or other person with the intent to cause harm. Violence often results from anger, frustration, or fear and occurs because the perpetrators believe that they are threatened or that their opinion is right and the victim is wrong. Violence may occur suddenly without warning or following aggressive behavior. Violence can result in death or severe injury if the individual attacks a fellow individual or staff member.
- Aggression is the communication of a threat or intended act of violence and often occurs before an act of violence. This communication can occur verbally or nonverbally. Gestures, shouting, speaking increasingly loudly, invasion of personal space, or prolonged eye contact are examples of aggression, requiring that the individual be redirected or removed from the situation.

Managing Aggressive or Violent Behavior

Managing aggressive or violent behavior is an important skill for the sleep technologist who may encounter patients who exhibit this behavior, especially patients with severe mental illness or dementia. When possible, a family member or caregiver should remain with patients at risk for violent outbursts. Medications may be prescribed to calm patients, but these may affect the polysomnogram. Other strategies include the following:

Reducing perceived threat	Do not make direct eye contact.
	Leave doors open, and do not block exits.
	Reassure patients.
Defusing the situation	Avoid conflict by deflecting rather than reacting.
	Remain nonjudgmental, passive, and allow patient to vent.
	Address situation directly by saying, "Your shouting is frightening me."
	Distract by offering food or drink.
Preventing injury or attack	Maintain a safe distance from patient, that is, out of the striking zone.

	Face the patient at all times.
	Remain alert for possible violent acts.
	Call for assistance or security if necessary.

Sleep Deprivation and Night-Shift Workers

Night-shift workers are at increased risk for sleep deprivation and often cannot change working hours, which would be the ideal solution. Other interventions include:

- Sleep extra hours on days off (at least 2 days/week).
- Avoid working more than 12–16 hours at one time.
- Monitor personal levels of alertness and impairment to increase safety.
- Avoid drinking alcohol, which can increase sleepiness and impairment.
- Avoid driving between 2 am and 9 am when most people are least alert.
- Take a 45-minute or 2-hour nap before beginning the night shift.
- Increase lighting at work to promote alertness.
- Drink caffeinated drinks, such as coffee, 1 hour before a period of decreased alertness or increased sleepiness and stop ingestion at least 3 hours before sleep time as it may further impair sleeping.
- Use Modafinil (prescription drug) to decrease sleepiness during the night (similar in effect to amphetamines but with fewer side effects).

Sleep Technology Abbreviations

Common abbreviations used for sleep technology include the following:

AI	Apnea index
AHI	Apnea-hypopnea index
CAP	Cyclic alternating pattern
EDS	Excessive daytime sleepiness
EPAP	Expiratory positive airway pressure
IEA	Interictal epileptiform activity
IPAP	Inspiratory positive airway pressure
Non-REM	Non-rapid eye movement
OA	Obstructive apnea
OH	Obstructive hypopnea
OSAS	Obstructive sleep apnea syndrome
OSA/H	Obstructive sleep apnea-hypopnea
PLMS	Periodic limb movements in sleep
PRC	Phase response curve
PSG	Polysomnogram
RBD	REM behavior disorder
RDI	Respiratory disturbance index
REM	Rapid eye movement
RERA	Respiratory effort-related arousals
RLS	Restless legs syndrome
SAH	Sleep apnea-hypopnea
SE	Sleep efficiency
SOL	Sleep onset latency
SWS	Short-wave sleep

SPT	Sleep period time
TST	Total sleep time
TSP	Total sleep period
TWT	Total wake time
WASO	Wake-after-sleep onset

Determining Treatment Interventions and Selecting and Fitting Masks and Interfaces

Interfaces

Interfaces are used with noninvasive ventilation to deliver pressurized air to the patient rather than intubation or tracheostomy. Patients may need to try various interfaces to find one that is effective and comfortable. A number of different types of interfaces are available, all which are secured by straps or headgear.

- Nasal mask: This mask fits over the nose but not into the nares. This is useful for patients who are nasal breathers, but the danger of air leaks exists if people breathe through their mouths or are edentulous and if continuous positive airway pressure is high. Risk of aspiration is low because the mouth is free.
- Oral mask: This mask fits only over the mouth but is rarely used.
- Orofacial mask: The orofacial mask covers the nose and mouth area but usually leaves the eyes free; however, the risk of aspiration is increased. There is more dead space than with a nasal mask, and there is an increased risk of leakage as well as claustrophobia.
- Nasal pillow: This mask has "pillows," often made of soft silicone, which fit into each nostril, providing a seal while leaving the bridge of the nose and the mouth exposed. This mask easily dislodges and may dry and irritate nasal passages, but it is less claustrophobic.

Nasal Pillows

Nasal pillows are fitted after the patient's nostrils are examined because the pillows that fit into the patient's nostrils are round. If the patient has slot-shaped nostrils, it may be impossible to get an airtight fit, and the pillows may cause pressure and pain. Additionally, some people have different-sized nostrils, so each nostril may need a separate size.

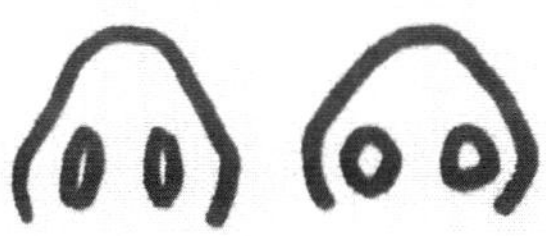

Typically, women use small-to-medium nasal pillows, and men, medium-to-large pillows. Nasal pillows must fit snugly into each nostril because if they are too loose, air will leak. A lubricant (e.g., Ayr) may provide some comfort. Once the pillow size is selected and pillows are attached to the nose piece, the swivel piece is attached, using an angle adapter if necessary; the air hose is positioned midline between the eyes, downward, or to the right or left, depending on the patient's usual sleeping position. The headgear or straps are adjusted to fit. Straps should be snug but not constrictive. One or two fingers should easily slide under the secured strap.

Nasal Masks

Nasal masks for noninvasive positive pressure ventilation fit over the nose, but the mouth is left free, so nasal masks are not effective for mouth breathers or those who are edentulous. There are many different nasal masks available, so the manufacturer's instructions must be examined before fitting. The piece that fits over the nose is typically soft and made of silicone or a gel material so that it adheres to the skin without causing undue pressure. The nose must be examined to make sure it fits easily into the nasal cup and is not compressed. Any forehead pad must be adjusted so that it is comfortably in the middle of the forehead. The angle between the nose and the forehead is adjusted with the stability adjuster. The headgear and straps are tightened and secured so they fit snuggly while not constricting (allowing one to two fingers to slip beneath straps). The airflow tube is positioned, using the swivel piece, to the most convenient position, depending on the patient's usual sleeping position.

Orofacial Masks

Orofacial masks are often more effective than nasal masks because both the nose and mouth are covered; however, there is an increase in dead space and an increased risk of aspiration. Additionally, some patients become claustrophobic, and orofacial masks are often more uncomfortable for the patient, so it must be adjusted carefully.

- Check the size of the mask against the patient's face to ensure that it will cover from above the nose to below the mouth.
- Loosen the straps or headgear and pull them over the head while moving the mask forward and positioning it over nose and mouth. The soft silicone of the rim should mold against the skin.
- Adjust straps or headgear so that the mask is securely against the face but not excessively tight.
- Check the forehead angle to ensure that there is no excess pressure on the bridge of the nose.
- Attach the swivel piece and tubing, and position the tubing to the most convenient position, depending on the patient's usual sleeping position.

Oral Masks

Oral masks are appropriate for people with nasal congestion and other nasal obstruction that cause them to breathe primarily through the mouth. Most oral masks have a soft silicone insert that goes inside the mouth and a retractable cover on the outside as well as straps to hold the appliance in place. Steps to application include:

- Fasten the straps to one side of the appliance.
- Connect the flexible tubing.
- Pull back the retractable outside cover to expose the mouthpiece.
- Insert the mouthpiece, one side at a time, into the mouth between the teeth and the cheeks.
- Ask the patient to move the lips back comfortably over the mouthpiece.
- Snap the cover back over the mouth.
- Fasten the straps around the head and adjust to secure the mask.
- Examine the nostrils for shape and size and insert nasal plugs. Nasal plugs should be used with the mask for at least the first few weeks if the patient does any nasal breathing.

PROBLEM-SOLVING

Claustrophobia: Claustrophobia with any interface is common among patients, especially full facemasks, and this anxiety may further impair breathing and cause the patient to feel short of breath. In this case, patients may need time to adjust.

- Ask the patient to practice holding the mask in position without straps or tubing connected, suggesting that the patient read or watch television as a distraction. Encourage patients to pull the mask away from the face if it becomes uncomfortable, deep breathe, and then reposition the mask.
- As the patient becomes more comfortable, follow the same procedure with air flowing through the mask but no straps or headgear. Again, encourage the patient to pull the mask away if it becomes uncomfortable.
- Once the patient can accept airflow, turn off the airflow, attach straps or headgear, and ask the patient to practice wearing the mask while secured. Again, allow the patient to remove the headgear and mask as necessary.
- Last, apply the mask with airflow and headgear in place, but allow the patient to control the duration of treatment until anxiety recedes.
- Allow as many repetitions as necessary.

Noise and air hunger: Noise can interfere with sleep by distracting patients and their partners even though the new machines are much quieter than earlier versions. Most people adapt to the noise over time. Patient solutions include:

- Earplugs
- White noise machines
- Soft classical music

For short periods during the daytime, patients can be told to listen to the machine to get used to the sound.

Air hunger is when some patients feel short of breath while using positive airway pressure. Solutions include:

- Examine the mask and tubing for an air leak and correct.
- With ramp pressure, increase beginning pressure as it may be set too low. If using automatic positive air pressure, consult the physician about increasing the starting pressure.
- Use a chinstrap to keep the mouth closed if using a nasal appliance and the mouth is open during sleep, or switch to an orofacial mask.

Air leaks in face masks: Air leaks in face masks may occur in spite of the fact that orofacial and nasal masks generally have soft silicone rims that mold to the face; however, if the straps are too tight or the skin is very wrinkled, creases can occur that allow air leaks. Masks often become unseated during the night and leak. Solutions include:

- Reposition the mask by pulling it forward away from the face for 2–3 seconds and then reseat it. Repeat as necessary. This is often sufficient if leaks occur during the night with patient movement.
- Loosen headgear or straps if they are too tight as this can increase the chance of creasing of the skin.
- Apply the mask with airflow turned on as this helps establish a seal.

- Observe the patient carefully during sleep to determine if the airflow tube is positioned correctly for the patient's preferred sleep position as the tube can dislodge the mask.
- Change to a different type or size of interface if leaks persist.

Air swallowing and eye irritation: Air swallowing can cause burping on awakening and abdominal distention in some patients because some of the pressurized air flows down the esophagus instead of into the lungs. Solutions include:

- Double the pillow under the patient's head to bring the head forward and the chin toward the chest (about a 45° angle) as this position closes off the esophagus. This usually relieves air swallowing for most patients.
- Observe the patient carefully to ensure a change in head position does not impair breathing.
- In some cases, lower pressure settings by small increments and evaluate.

Eye irritation almost always relates to air leaks and air blowing across the eyes. Solutions include:

- Examine all masks for leaks.
- Reseat or adjust mask fitting as necessary.
- Check straps to make sure they are secure but not too tight.
- Change to a different type or size of mask if other solutions are ineffective.

Nasal irritation or dryness and skin irritation: Nasal irritation or dryness sometimes associated with nosebleeds is a common complaint with positive airway pressure, especially with nasal pillows because they are placed inside the nostrils. Solutions include:

- Check the shape and size of the nostrils to ensure that the correct-sized nasal pillows are used for each nostril.
- Use lubricant (e.g., Ayr) during insertion of nasal pillows.
- Increase humidification to reduce dryness.
- Change to a different type of mask if irritation continues.

A rash, skin irritation, or pressure sores may develop in some patients where the mask contacts the skin or beneath the mask. Solutions include:

- Check the headgear or straps to ensure they are not too tight.
- Instruct the patient to clean the mask each day before use, and observe the patient doing so.
- Make sure the mask is thoroughly dry before applying.
- Provide cushioning protection for pressure sores when applying the mask.
- Refer to a physician for evaluation of possible allergies or the need for medication for a skin rash.
- Consider changing to a different type of mask if other solutions fail.

Mouth breathing and mouth leaks: Mouth breathing and mouth leaks can exacerbate dryness of the mucous membranes and lead to a reduction in pressure as some of the pressurized air leaks out of the mouth. Additionally, mouth breathing can result in collapse of the upper airways, increasing airway obstruction so that treatment is ineffective for obstructive sleep apnea syndrome. Solutions include:

- Adjust pressure settings and observe for a response.
- Evaluate for nasal congestion or a deviated septum, and refer to a physician for treatment.
- Increase the temperature of heated humidification to relieve nasal irritation and congestion.

- Try a chinstrap to keep the mouth closed (although air can still leak out between the lips).
- Use positive airway pressure with expiratory pressure relief or heated humidifier tubing.
- Change to a full orofacial mask if necessary.
- If the sleeping position is supine, try a supported side-lying position as this may relieve mouth breathing for some patients.
- Do not tape the mouth shut as this can lead to aspiration or asphyxiation.

Chronic fatigue or sleepiness: Chronic fatigue or sleepiness in patients should show improvement using positive airway pressure (PAP), but sometimes persistent sleepiness occurs despite treatments. Solutions include the following:

- Give the patient time to adjust to the machine as not all patients see results immediately.
- Evaluate the patient's total sleep time (TST) to ensure it is 7 hours a day or more, and ask about daytime napping, which must be included in TST.
- Check the mask for leaks as inadequate pressure may result in apnea and poor sleep quality.
- Review symptoms associated with a poorly fitted mask or mouth breathing, such as dry mouth, sore nasal passages, and dry eyes.
- Review sleep hygiene with patient.
- Discuss habits related to alcohol, caffeine, and cigarettes before bed as these may impair sleeping.
- Evaluate environmental factors, such as temperature, noise, bed partners, or interruptions.
- Ask about restless legs syndrome or bruxism as these may interfere with sleep.
- Observe the patient during sleep to determine if the PAP device remains in place throughout the night.
- Reassess the type of mask used.

Positive Airway Pressure Devices

Continuous positive airway pressure (CPAP) can be delivered by a wide range of equipment, starting with the most basic, relatively inexpensive machines to expensive computerized equipment. All positive airway pressure devices have an air blower that delivers pressurized room air to an interface or mask. Pressure can be increased or decreased by adjusting the speed or the amount of airflow, with most machines generating pressure ranging from 2–20 cm H_2O. Carbon dioxide is expelled through a vent or nonrebreather. These may be large or small, but all have filters in the back and can be used with a variety of masks (e.g., oral, nasal, orofacial, nasal pillow). Some have built-in heated humidifiers, and all can be used with cool passover or heated humidifiers. Many basic machines do not adjust for environmental factors, such as altitude, and many do not have an internal memory to generate sleep reports. Some may switch between 110 and 220 volts. Even basic machines allow for a gradual rise to selected pressure. More sophisticated CPAP machines usually have software and downloadable memories that can provide reports regarding respiratory events. Altitude compensation is usually automatic.

Bilevel positive airway pressure (Bi-PAP, BiPAP ST, auto BiPAP) devices deliver two levels of pressure, which can be preset. Inspiratory positive airway pressure (IPAP) is set at a higher level than expiratory airway pressure (EPAP). This allows for the pressure needed to open the airway during inspiration but reduces pressure to facilitate expiration. Typically, Bi-PAP devices do not compensate for altitude and can be used with humidification. Some have software and downloadable memory to generate reports of sleep events.

Bi-PAP ST (spontaneous-timed) devices have two pressure settings for each breath as well as settings for the number of respirations so that they can trigger inspiration if the respiratory rate falls below a preset level, an important consideration for central sleep apnea and other pulmonary disorders. Settings include a spontaneous mode, which triggers increased pressure after the person attempts to breathe, and a timed mode, which triggers increased pressure to initiate respiration within a preset time.

Auto Bi-PAP (auto-titrating) devices are also available and can vary both IPAP and EPAP automatically as needed to promote adequate ventilation.

Automatic positive airway pressure (APAP) devices have self-setting technology to determine the correct pressure for the individual patient and include software and downloadable memory for generation of reports about sleep events. Some machines require specific masks or nasal pillows, and they are not standardized as to settings or the type of reports generated, so the operation manual must be reviewed carefully. These machines are able to detect upper airway obstruction and adjust pressures to compensate. Pressure is adjusted for both inspiration and expiration. Because APAP adjusts automatically, it may be useful during titration in the sleep lab. APAP devices use different sensors, such as vibration sensors to detect snoring and can identify episodes of apnea and hypopnea. APAP devices are set by technicians (according to a physician's prescription) within a range, usually 3–4 cm H_2O and 18–20 cm H_2O.

Adaptive servoventilation devices provide a baseline positive airway pressure and breathing assist to ensure adequate ventilation (at a preset level) with each breath to 90% of average for the patient.

Titrating Positive Airway Pressure and Oxygen and Troubleshooting

Testing with a Polysomnogram

Testing with a polysomnogram (PSG) is usually done before positive airway pressure (PAP) is titrated to determine the type of sleep disorder and the need for PAP. This is done in one of two ways:

- Two-day testing: The first day of testing involves a nocturnal PSG for diagnosis. If obstructive sleep apnea (OSA) is found, then the patient returns for another night during which continuous PAP titration is completed to determine adequate settings to control apnea.
- Split-night testing: This testing uses the first half of the night for a diagnostic PSG. If a clear pattern of OSA is present (≥ 40 apneas–hypopneas in 2 hours or an apnea-hypopnea index of 20–40 with significant oxygen desaturation during this period) or if a diagnosis of OSA has already been made, titration is done in the second half of the night (at least 3 hours). This testing may be used for both the initial diagnosis and follow-up to determine the persistence of symptoms and the effectiveness of treatment.

Demonstration

Demonstration of continuous positive airway pressure (CPAP) with a nasal mask should be given to patients before titration so that they are comfortable with the equipment and understand how it functions.

- Two-day testing: The demonstration can take place on the second day of testing before sleep.
- Split-night testing: Usually a presumptive diagnosis of obstructive sleep apnea (OSA) has been made, so the demonstration is done before sleep, anticipating that CPAP titration will occur during the second half of the night.

The initial demonstration should include:

- An explanation of the physiological changes during OSA and how they affect oxygen levels and breathing.
- An explanation of the parameters of OSA, which are usually 15 periods of apnea or more, lasting 10 sec/min or more, an arousal demonstration by an electroencephalogram shift (≥ 3 seconds), or a drop in oxygen saturation (SpO2) by 3%–4%.
- Fitting of the mask, headgear, and straps so that they can be easily and quickly applied during the night.
- Practice wearing the mask with and without air pressure.
- An explanation of the titration process.

CPAP Titration

Continuous positive airway pressure (CPAP) titration attempts to find the correct pressure that prevents episodes of apnea when they are most severe, usually when the patient is lying supine during REM sleep; this position promotes collapse of the upper airway, which worsens with REM-associated atonia.

Equipment preparation	Fill humidifier with fresh distilled water (tap water may erode heating element) to maximum fill line.
	Program the machine with the person's setting or set the pressure dial, depending on the type of machine.
	Check the filter to make sure it is in place and clean.
	Set parameters for the ramp button, low pressure to high, and time to maximum (usually 45 minutes). (This function is usually not used during the initial titration.)
Patient preparation	Fit the mask, headgear, and straps. Release straps on one side only so that the mask can be applied quickly without fitting during the night if titration occurs during split-night testing.
	Provide a demonstration of the mask with and without air (even if patient has had a previous demonstration). Apply electrodes and sensors for polysomnography.

Continuous positive airway pressure (CPAP) titration begins with equipment preparation and patient preparation. Additional steps include the following:

Problem anticipation	During the demonstration, ask the patient to open the mouth while receiving positive airway pressure (PAP) so the patient can experience a mouth leak. Keeping the mouth open is usually uncomfortable, making it easier to keep the mouth closed.
	Loosen the mask to break the seal during PAP so the patient can experience an air leak (usually felt as air in the eyes or on the face or heard as a whistling or whooshing sound).
	Demonstrate unsnapping the tube and unfastening leads, and ask the patient to practice so the patient can get up to urinate during the night without removing the mask.
	Tell the patient that she or he may feel somewhat uncomfortable with PAP at first but to just relax and try to breathe normally.
	Reassure the patient that it may take longer than normal to fall asleep (? 30 minutes) at first.

Continuous positive airway pressure (CPAP) titration begins when the CPAP equipment is set, the patient is prepared, and anticipated problems discussed. Titration procedures may vary somewhat, according to the manufacturer's guidelines and sleep center policies.

Titration

- Begin CPAP treatment when the patient is ready for sleep.
- Begin with pressure at the lowest setting, usually 5 cm H2O, and maintain this low pressure until the patient falls asleep.
- Check the polysomnographic tracings, and watch the patient for position and signs of snoring, mouth leaks, or air leaks.
- Increase positive airway pressure 1 cm H2O at a time at set intervals, usually about every 15 minutes, and observe effects, including changes in oxygen saturation, electroencephalogram, electromyogram, and electrocardiogram.
- Ensure that the patient is supine and in REM sleep for part of the titration period, or position patient in the supine position for sleep.
- Adjust the pressure up or down as indicated until the optimal level is reached, indicated by the absence of periods of apnea, hypopnea, respiratory effort–related arousals, oxygen desaturation, and other sleep disordered breathing, such as snoring.

Apnea–Hypopnea Index and Upper Airway Resistance Syndrome

Apnea-hypopnea index (AHI)	AHI is the total of apneic and hypopneic events in 1 hour of sleep. Apnea is absence of breathing while hypopnea is ineffectual or inadequate breathing, with exchange of air about 25%–70% of normal. The AHI for obstructive sleep apnea (OSA) is 15 or more.

Upper airway resistance syndrome (UARS)	UARS is characterized by an AHI of 5 or less but with increased numbers of respiratory effort-related arousals (RERAs) because of airway resistance to breathing during sleep caused by small, restricted airways. While snoring is a common indicator of upper airway collapse and OSA, the elimination of apneic periods and snoring alone does not indicate adequate titration for UARS. Rather, the focus must be on elimination of RERAs as well because some patients, especially women, have UARS without snoring. The oronasal thermistors normally used to evaluate airflow may not be sufficient to diagnose RERAs in UARS because RERAs may be less obvious; instead, esophageal cannulas with pressure transducers may be needed to show a reduction in flow.

Respiratory Effort–Related Arousals and Respiratory Disturbance Index

Respiratory effort-related arousals (RERAs)	RERAs typically occur when the patient falls asleep and begins snoring as muscle tone decreases, allowing the upper airway to collapse. The central nervous system senses apnea and responds by increasing muscle tone, blood pressure, and the metabolic rate. These changes cause the person to arouse enough to trigger inspiration, at which point the patient usually falls back to sleep. RERAs may occur many times during the night, preventing the person from falling into a deep sleep and resulting in chronic sleepiness.
Respiratory disturbance index (RDI)	RDI is the total of all respiratory disturbance events, including apnea and hypopnea as well as snoring, arousals, desaturation, and hypoventilation in 1 hour. In some cases, the apnea-hypopnea index and the RDI may be identical, but in other cases the RDI will be higher. The RDI is used to determine the severity of sleeping disorders: Normal: < 5 Mild: 5–20 Moderate: 20–40 Severe: > 40

Adverse Effects

Positive airway pressure (PAP) therapy can cause a number of adverse effects, some because of the equipment but others because of pressure settings or social issues. Compliance (using for 4 hours or more a night 70% or more of the time) depends on identifying adverse effects and helping the patient to find solutions:

- If PAP is inadequately humidified:
  - Nasal irritation - Dryness and congestion; Watery discharge; Bleeding
- Excess pressure
  - Air leaks and mouth leaks
  - Air swallowing and difficulty exhaling
  - Discomfort in chest
  - Conjunctivitis (related to air leaks)
  - Increased arousals and difficulty sleeping
  - Barotrauma (lung damage): rare and usually related to blockage of exhalation valve with no pressure release valve or airway pressure alarm; sometimes results in pneumothorax or pneumoencephaly

- Mask
    - Skin irritation
    - Rash
    - Ulcerations (usually related to excess pressure or improperly sized mask)
    - Allergic reaction
- Social reactions
    - Partner conflict
    - Inconvenience
    - Resistance to treatment

REM Latency, Sleep Efficiency, and Sleep Onset Latency

Effects of positive airway pressure on sleep must be evaluated.

REM latency	REM latency	This is the time period from the first epoch of sleep until the onset of REM sleep.
Sleep efficiency	SE	SE is calculated by comparing the percentage of time spent sleeping to the time spent in bed. If a person sleeps 4 hours and spends 8 hours in bed, the ratio is 4:8, and the SE is 50%. Formula: Total sleep time X 100/total sleep period.
Sleep onset latency	SOL	SOL determines the amount of time needed to go from an awake state to a sleep state. SOL is used with the multiple latency sleep test to judge the severity of sleepiness during the day: 0–5 minutes: severe 5–10 minutes: moderate 10–15 minutes: mild 15–20 minutes: normal SOL is also monitored during nocturnal polysomnography, with normal SOL about 10–15 minutes.

Sleep Period Time, Total Sleep Time, Total Sleep Period, Total Wake Time, and Wake-After-Sleep Onset

Effects of positive airway pressure on sleep must be evaluated.

Sleep period time	SPT	The SPT is calculated as the percentage of total time spent at different sleep stages. Thus, if 22% of sleep time was spent in REM sleep, the report would read "REM, 22% SPT."
Total sleep time	TST	TST is total sleep in minutes for all stages of sleep (stage 1, 2, and 3 non-REM and REM).
Total sleep period	TSP	TSP begins with lights out and ends with lights on and is calculated in hours and minutes. (also sometimes referred to as total bedtime time or TBT).
Total wake time	TWT	TWT is the total number of minutes awake in the TSP (lights out to lights on).
Wake-after-sleep onset	WASO	WASO is the total minutes spent awake after first falling asleep and until the final awakening time.

APAP Titration

Automatic positive airway pressure (APAP) titration is sometimes used for the initial positive airway titration. While machines vary, generally they are able to detect upper airway obstruction, limitations in airflow associated with snoring, and apneas-hypopneas, with a variety of different types of built-in sensors. For example, some machines require special masks with vibration sensors that detect snoring. When obstruction occurs that limits airflow, the APAP device increases the pressure until the obstruction resolves. Then, the pressure is slowly reduced until the obstruction recurs, thus determining the correct pressure. Not all APAP devices are able to differentiate between apneas and hypopneas, and some may not identify obstruction not related to snoring. The technologist should carefully review data to determine the effectiveness of APAP settings. Additionally, APAP titration levels cannot always be safely applied to continuous positive airway pressure (CPAP), so the effectiveness of the pressure setting with CPAP should be evaluated separately. APAP is contraindicated for congestive heart failure, chronic obstructive pulmonary disease, and obesity-hypoventilation syndrome, central apneas, and previous surgery of upper airway.

PAP for Home Titration/Treatment

Home titration and treatment of sleep disorders have become more common as automatic positive airway pressure (APAP) devices have become readily available and sophisticated; physicians have begun to send patients who have a presumptive diagnosis of obstructive sleep apnea syndrome home with APAP or continuous positive airway (CPAP) devices to self-titrate and treat, often with minimal instructions and no diagnostic polysomnography. Considerations include:

- Patients with CPAP may set pressures to low to be effective or too high, increasing sleeping disorders and sometimes causing central sleep apnea.
- Patients or partners typically use snoring as an indicator of symptom relief, but relieving snoring alone may not resolve apnea-hypopnea issues.
- Diagnosis by guessing is not an effective method of diagnosing sleep disorders, as the presumptive diagnosis may be incorrect.
- Selected patients with APAP may be able to use the machine in the home environment for titrating, but the data should then be reviewed by a sleep technologist to determine if the settings are optimal for the patient or if further testing or treatment is indicated.

Differences Between Continuous and Automatic Airway Pressure

The differences between continuous (CPAP) and automatic (APAP) airway pressures have been evaluated by a number of small studies with the following results:

- Apnea-hypopnea (AHI): Both CPAP and APAP are equally effective in reducing AHI.
- Oxygen saturation (SpO2): SpO2 improves with both CPAP and APAP, but APAP is associated with a slightly lower average saturation level.
- Sleep effectiveness: Both CPAP and APAP are effective in improving the quality of sleep, including reducing arousals and increasing REM sleep. Patients requiring high pressures to prevent obstructive sleep apneas (OSAs) usually find sleep quality is better with APAP.
- Daytime sleepiness (Epworth Sleepiness Score): APAP and CPAP are generally similar, but some patients, especially those whose OSA is dependent on body position or stage of sleep, rate APAP higher.
- Airway pressure: Average airway pressure is lower with APAP than CPAP because of pressure variability.
- Patient compliance: Overall compliance is similar with APAP and CPAP.

C-Flex and EPR

Two intermediary devices, C-Flex and EPR, between continuous airway pressure (CPAP) and bilevel positive airway pressure (Bi-PAP) may improve compliance because some patients cannot tolerate CPAP because of the pressure during exhalation; this often results in discontinuation of treatments or poor compliance.

- C-Flex (by Respironics) is an expiratory pressure relief device and is a modified CPAP machine that has some elements of Bi-PAP. It provides a steady inspiratory pressure but allows patients to select a reduction in pressure during expiration in the range of 1–3 cm H2O. C-Flex monitors airflow, triggering the short pressure reduction when it detects a change to indicate exhalation. The amount of pressure reduction varies slightly with each breath, depending on airflow.
- EPR (by ResMed), another expiratory pressure relief device, provides similar relief of pressure during exhalation but does so by reducing motor speed.

Bilevel Positive Airway Pressure

Indications for bilevel positive airway pressure (Bi-PAP), also referred to as noninvasive positive pressure ventilation (NPPV), rather than continuous positive airway pressure (CPAP), include the following:

- Continuous positive airway pressure (CPAP) intolerance - If the pressure needed to control obstructive sleep apnea (OSA) is high, the patient may have difficulty with expiration (smothering) and may have air leaks, mouth leaks, and difficulty tolerating treatment. Some patients still have difficulty if expiratory positive airway pressure (EPAP) is set too high. Patients who cannot control OSA with CPAP may achieve control with Bi-PAP.
- Central sleep apnea (CSA) - Because the central nervous system is not triggering respirations adequately, CSA does not always respond to CPAP alone. In that case, Bi-PAP ST (spontaneous-timed), which triggers respirations if apnea occurs, is used. Specific indications include all of the following:
  - OSA has been ruled out as the primary cause of apnea.
  - CPAP has not proven effective.
  - Oxygen saturation is 88% or less continuously for 5 minutes with the usual fraction of inspired oxygen.
  - Bi-PAP (with or without ST) demonstrates clinical improvement.
  - Bi-PAP does sometimes trigger CSA if the inspiratory positive airway pressure is set significantly higher than EPAP.
- **Chronic obstructive lung disease (COPD)** - Severe COPD may require Bi-PAP because of an impaired ability to ventilate. Specific indications include all of the following:
  - There is a PaCO2 of 52 mm Hg or more (awake and with the usual fraction of inspired oxygen [FIO2]).
  - The oxygen saturation (SpO2) is 88% or less continuously for 5 minutes at minimum of oxygen at 2 L/min.
  - Patient does not have obstructive sleep apnea, and CPAP treatment is not effective or ruled out.
  - Bi-PAP ST (spontaneous-timed) may be indicated if initial use of Bi-PAP alone is not adequate to control symptoms.
- **Neuromuscular diseases (NMDs)** - NMDs, such as amyotrophic lateral sclerosis, which are thoracic-restrictive, impair the ability to breathe. Specific indications include:

- The $PaCO_2$ is 45 mm Hg or more during waking hours with a normal FIO_2 for that patient.
- The SpO_2 is 88% or less continuously for 5 minutes.
- Maximal inspiratory pressure is 60 cm H_2O or less.
- Forced vital capacity is 50% or less of that expected for a patient with an NMD.

- **Heart failure (with pulmonary edema)** - Heart failure may seriously impact respirations and sleep. With pulmonary edema, the alveoli become compressed with fluid and collapsed so that oxygen–carbon dioxide exchange is impaired. During inspiration, the alveoli do not fill adequately, and they may completely collapse on expiration. Prolonged heart failure is often associated with weakening of the muscles of respiration. During sleep, when muscle activity is lessened, this can increase the symptoms of heart failure. Bi-PAP/NNPV may be indicated because inspiratory positive airway pressure helps to inflate the alveoli during inspiration, and expiratory positive airway pressure prevents collapse of the alveoli during expiration, promoting better air exchange and decreasing the need for supplementary oxygen. Additionally, as heart failure increases, muscle activity is impaired, so Bi-PAP ST (spontaneous-timed) may be needed to trigger respirations. This use is usually restricted to the hospital rather than at home.
- **Obesity- hypoventilation syndrome (OHS)** - OHS occurs when the body mass index is 30 kg/m^2 or more, resulting in impaired respirations, hypoxia, and hypercapnia during sleep. The obesity results in impairment of muscles of inspiration, restricting the thorax and causing hypoventilation, leading to hypercapnia. Most patients develop OHS with obstructive sleep apnea (OSA), characterized by five or more apneas–hypopneas an hour. About 10% of patients with OHS have primarily hypercapnia with an increase of 10 mm Hg during sleep. Medicare guidelines for treatment with Bi-PAP/NNPV rather than CPAP include:
  - Evidence of central apnea with a polysomnogram
  - An oxygen saturation of 88% or less, persisting for 5 minutes or more
  - With CPAP failure for OSA but a demonstrated improvement with Bi-PAP
  - Evidence of hypercapnia with OSA: awake $PaCO_2$ of 45 mm Hg or less

Titrating Bilevel Positive Airway Pressure

Bilevel positive airway pressure (Bi-PAP) titration begins with the same steps as continuous positive airway pressure (CPAP) titration, including educating the patient, mask fitting and application, and a demonstration with practice. Titration steps include the following:

- Set initial pressures
  - Expiratory positive airway pressure (EPAP): Usually set at 4 cm H_2O, but if the patient has had prior CPAP, then the EPAP may be set at the lowest pressure that opened the airway.
  - Inspiratory positive airway pressure (IPAP): Usually set at 8 cm H_2O or at least 4 cm H_2O above EPAP, although some technologists prefer to set the initial IPAP at 2 cm H_2O above EPAP.
- Evaluate
  - Response to the initial setting must be evaluated to determine if there is evidence of apnea, snoring, or obstruction. If symptoms are clear, then the initial setting may be adequate.

- Control apnea
    - Apneas are monitored and treated first, so if apneas and oxygen desaturation persist, then both the IPAP and EPAP are increased in 2 cm H2O increments every 5 minutes until apneic episodes stop.
    - In some cases, EPAP is increased only for obstructive sleep apneas.

Bilevel positive airway pressure (Bi-PAP) titration, after the initial instructions, demonstrations, initial pressures, evaluating, and controlling apnea, includes:

- Control hypopnea
    - Increase inspiratory positive airway pressure (IPAP) only by 1 cm H2O every 15–30 minutes until the apnea–hypopnea index (AHI) is less than 5 and hypopneas stop.
- Control desaturation
    - If desaturation persists after apneas and hypopneas are eliminated, continue to increase IPAP in 1 cm H2O increments.
    - If desaturation does not respond to increases in IPAP alone, increase both IPAP and expiratory positive airway pressure in 1 cm H2O increments.
    - If still no response or indications of excess pressure are evident, then stop the increase and adjust downward as necessary, but consider supplementary oxygen.
- Monitor snoring
    - If apneas and hypopneas are eliminated but snoring or limitations in flow persist, then check for air leaks. If a leak persists, reduce pressure until the leak stops, and then slowly increase pressure again until there are five or fewer apneas–hypopneas an hour.

Final monitoring steps with bilevel positive airway pressure (Bi-PAP) titration, after the optimal inspiratory (IPAP) and expiratory (EPAP) positive airway pressure settings are achieved, include the following:

- Observe REM sleep
    - Evaluate breathing patterns while the patient is in a supine position. If abnormalities occur, then increase IPAP and EPAP 1 cm H2O until abnormalities stop.
- Monitor for excess pressure
    - If central apneas begin to occur regularly (a sign of excess pressure), decrease IPAP only (maintaining at least a 4-cm H2O difference between IPAP and EPAP).
    - If the difference between IPAP and EPAP is less than 4 cm H2O or there is no response to a decrease in IPAP only, decrease both IPAP and EPAP.
- Control central sleep apneas (CSAs)
    - If CSAs begin to occur before the optimal setting to treat obstructive apnea, use a timed mode for Bi-PAP with backup respiratory rate, and decrease EPAP and IPAP to 2 cm H2O before the onset of CSAs; then increase IPAP only by 1–2 cm H2O until there are five or fewer apneas–hypopneas an hour.

With bilevel positive airway (Bi-PAP) titration, additional monitoring may be used. Carbon dioxide may be monitored as an indirect method to determine $PaCO_2$ and evidence of hypercapnia.

- PetCO2: Exhaled end-tidal carbon dioxide levels, using respiratory spectrometry or infrared spectrophotometry, are not always reliable during sleep so they are rarely used for adults but may be used with pediatric patients to observe for prolonged obstructive hypoventilation (a condition more common to infants and children).
- PtcCO2: Transcutaneous carbon dioxide monitoring, using a silver chloride electrode or infrared capnometer, likewise is used for pediatric polysomnography but is not always given an adequate estimation of PaCO2 for adults.

Monitor carbon dioxide	If using carbon dioxide monitoring and it is within normal limits, maintain the inspiratory and expiratory positive airway pressures (I:E) differential at 4–6 cm H_2O.
	If hypercapnia occurs, the I:E differential can increase.

Bilevel Positive Airway Pressure Titration Grading

Bilevel positive airway pressure (Bi-PAP) titration should completely eliminate all indications of sleep-associated breathing disorders, such as periods of apnea or hypopnea and arousals, but this goal may not be realistic, depending on the patient's condition and baseline apnea-hypopnea index (AHI) established through initial polysomnography. Grading of titration adequacy includes:

- Excellent: At least 5 AHI/hr or more and some periods of REM sleep uninterrupted by arousals
- Good: At least 10 AHI/hr or more or by 50% if baseline AHI is 15/hr or less
- Adequate: AHI decreased to 75% of baseline although still 10 AHI/hr or more (This is common with severe obstructive sleep apnea syndrome with high rates of AHI.)
- Inadequate: AHI more than 75% of baseline and 10–20 AHI/hr or more.

If Bi-PAP is not effective, then the addition of oxygen or more invasive ventilation may be indicated.

Sleep Studies

Sleep studies are classified as types 1–4, depending upon the montage and place of testing:

- Type 1: Nocturnal polysomnograms are completed in a sleep center. Type 1 sleep study must include at least twelve channels of information, including electroencephalogram (EEG), electrocardiogram (ECG), electrooculogram (EOG), electromyogram (EMG, both chin and limb), pulse oximetry, and respiratory effort and airflow sensors. Type 1 is used to diagnose obstructive sleep apnea syndrome (OSAS) as well as other sleep disorders.
- Types 2, 3, and 4 are modified home sleep studies, using portable devices. These types are appropriate only for OSAS because they provide limited information and are unattended.
  - Type 2 must include at least seven channels of information: EEG, ECG, EOG, EMG, pulse oximetry, respiratory effort, and airflow sensors.
  - Type 3 must include at least three channels of information: one ECG lead to monitor heart rate, pulse oximetry, and two sensors for respiratory effort and airflow.
  - Type 4 must include one to three channels of information, including airflow and respiratory effort sensors.

Respiratory System During the Awake Stage

The respiratory system during the awake stage is under primary control of the autonomic nervous system. However, speaking and eating can interfere with respirations, and they can also be controlled voluntarily, such as when a person holds his or her breath. The upper respiratory tract, including the nose, nasal passages, sinuses, pharynx, tonsils, adenoids, larynx, and trachea, warms, filters, and moistens the air that is inhaled, but obstruction of the upper respiratory tract may interfere with this function and cause people to become mouth breathers. While breathing through the mouth occurs with exercise, chronic mouth breathing can cause dryness of the mucous membranes in the mouth and can result in abnormalities of facial growth in children. The lower respiratory tract (the lungs) accomplishes gas exchange, that is, oxygen for carbon dioxide.

Respiratory Terminology for Lung Volumes and Capacity

Respiratory terminology for lung volumes and lung capacities includes the following:

Tidal volume	Amount of air exchange with each breath (500 mL/kg for adults or 5–10 mL/kg for infants and children).
Residual volume	Amount of air remaining in the lungs after a forced exhalation. Average for adults is 1200 mL, but this may increase with chronic obstructive pulmonary disease (COPD).
Vital capacity	The maximal amount of air exhaled after maximal inhalation. Average for adults is 4600 mL; it decreases with neuromuscular disease, atelectasis, and fatigue.
Functional residual capacity	The amount of air remaining in the lungs after a normal exhalation; the average for adults is 2300 mL, but this may increase with COPD and decrease with acute respiratory distress syndrome.
Total lung capacity	The amount of air in the lungs after a maximal inhalation.
	Average for adults is 5800 mL, but this may increase with COPD and decrease with pneumonia or atelectasis.

Respiratory System During Stages 1, 2, and 3 Non-REM Sleep

The respiratory system during stages 1, 2, and 3 non-REM sleep is completely under the control of the autonomic nervous system and is not impacted by activities of the awake state; thus, respirations should become very regular in both the respiratory rate and the amplitude:

- Stages 1 and 2: Some periodic breathing (irregular respirations with brief periods of apnea–hypopnea) may occur at sleep onset and throughout stage 1 but should disappear by stage 2. Periodic breathing is common with congestive heart failure.
- Stage 3: Respirations should remain regular with some decrease noted in tidal volume and functional residual capacity as well as a decrease in minute ventilation. $PaCO2$ increases, and $PaO2$ decreases. Inspiratory airflow decreases, and upper airway resistance increases. Muscle activity (muscles of respiration) decreases.

Respiratory System During REM Sleep

The respiratory system during REM sleep changes as respirations become much more irregular in rate, amplitude, and tidal volume. Periodic breathing or central apneas (10–30 seconds) may occur during phasic REM sleep. Muscle hypotonia/atonia may affect the muscles of respiration, including the intercostals, and this can increase hypoventilation in patients with pulmonary disorders. The diaphragm muscle remains innervated by phrenic motor neurons, so it can compensate for the loss of other muscle function; however, if the diaphragm is impaired, such as with neuromuscular disease, then hypoventilation occurs. The $PaCO_2$ increases by 2–5 mm Hg while the PaO_2 and functional residual capacity decrease, increasing hypoxemia in patients with sleep-disordered breathing because the compensatory ventilatory response is depressed. Upper airway resistance increases during REM sleep and can lead to collapse of the airway and obstructive sleep apnea syndrome.

SNORING

Snoring results from vibration within the respiratory system, often within the throat or nasal passages. The sound arises from the tissues vibrating against each other. Causes can include the following:

- Throat muscle weakness
- Obesity
- Nasal obstruction
- Tissues touching
- Drug use (alcohol or other muscle relaxant drugs)
- Supine position (The tongue may obstruct the airway.)

Snoring increases during sleep because the muscles relax, causing partial closure of the airway. Usually, the more the restriction in airflow, the louder the snoring. If related to nasal obstruction only (primary), snoring is usually regular and periodic and may be soft to loud. While annoying, this type of snoring is not a threat to health. Snoring related to obstructive sleep apnea is more irregular in rhythm and interrupted by periods of apnea-hypopnea and brief arousals. Patients may complain of headache on arising and chronic drowsiness.

CARDIOVASCULAR SYSTEM DURING SLEEP

The cardiovascular system during sleep responds to the control of both the sympathetic and parasympathetic nervous systems, causing changes in heart rate and blood pressure, although stroke volume usually remains constant with the lowest cardiac output during the final REM cycle. The changes can cause cardiovascular ischemia in some individuals:

- Stages 1, 2, and 3 non-REM sleep: For most patients, the parasympathetic nervous system is primary, causing a decrease in both the heart rate and blood pressure (decreased peripheral vascular resistance) by 5%–15%.
- REM sleep: During the phasic stage of REM sleep, the sympathetic nervous system affects the cardiovascular system by increasing both the heart rate and blood pressure (increased peripheral vascular resistance). However, during tonic REM sleep, the parasympathetic nervous system again lowers the heart rate, sometimes to bradycardic levels, and blood pressure.
- Arousal response: The sympathetic nervous system is involved in arousals, increasing heart rate and blood pressure.

GASTROINTESTINAL TRACT DURING SLEEP

The gastrointestinal tract during sleep slows down as a protective mechanism to prevent aspiration. Less saliva is produced, esophageal motility decreases, and the patient swallows less; however, the production of gastric acid increases during the night (peaking from 10 pm to 2 am) in response to stimulation of the parasympathetic nervous system. Stomach emptying slows during sleep. These changes pose a problem for patients with gastroesophageal reflux disease (GERD) because the increased acid flows back into the esophagus at the same time that clearance of secretions in the esophagus slows. This increases the risk of obstructive sleep apnea. Arousal, in turn, stimulates swallowing. Gastric slow waves decrease during stages 1, 2, and 3 non-REM sleep but not in REM sleep, resulting in fewer episodes of GERD during REM sleep. Pain or discomfort related to gastrointestinal disorders can disrupt sleep significantly. It is likely that GERD will increase during sleep if the patient lies in the right lateral decubitus position.

Compressed Oxygen

Oxygen can be supplied in a variety of different forms.

Compressed oxygen	Tanks of compressed oxygen are typically color-coded as white or green, although contents always need to be verified by checking the label on the tank. Tanks are labeled USP and Oxygen in a yellow diamond. Typical sizes include the following: H tanks, which are tall tanks (about 4.5 feet) E tanks, which are small portable tanks for short duration use Oxygen is under pressure, so tanks require a regulator, which includes the following: Cylinder valve, which turns the flow of oxygen on or off Pressure reducing valve, which reduces cylinder pressure (2200 psi) to 50 psi Flowmeter (with humidifier), which controls the liter per minute flow of oxygen to the patient The flowmeter is usually directly attached to a bubble jet humidifier to humidify the oxygen.

Liquid Oxygen

Oxygen can be supplied in a variety of different forms. Liquid oxygen (LOX) is stored at temperatures of –183°C in special cryogenic containers with 1 cubic foot of liquid oxygen equal to 860 cubic feet of oxygen gas. Small 4-pound tanks can be attached to a belt about a person's waist and may last up to 8 hours. One problem is that as the tanks slowly warm, the oxygen evaporates, losing as much as a half liter overnight. LOX is maintained at 21 psi, and tanks continuously vent, so they should be used in well-ventilated areas. Small tanks are usually refilled from a larger liquid oxygen reservoir tank, but touching the fill valve can result in burns. The weight of the tank is used to estimate the amount of oxygen remaining rather than pressure, so it is more difficult to determine the amount remaining.

Concentrated Oxygen

Oxygen can be supplied in a variety of different forms. Concentrators are portable electric devices that filter ambient air to produce oxygen. They are useful only for low-flow oxygen (usually 1–6 L/min) at lower concentrations (ranging from 50%–95%) although some larger devices are able to provide 10 L/min. Concentrators are frequently used for people who need at-home oxygen because they are relatively inexpensive compared to compressed or liquid oxygen. Concentrators are adequate for people who need supplemental rather than pure oxygen, such as those with sleep apnea. Small portable units that can be battery-powered are also available. Concentrators may be used in some sleep centers as well if a central oxygen supply is not available.

Safety Precautions for Use of Oxygen

Safety precautions for use of oxygen include the following:

- Avoid using combustible materials (e.g., oils, lotions, sprays) in the presence of oxygen, including collodion.
- Prohibit smoking, matches, or other flame-producing devices near oxygen.
- Secure tanks in an upright position to prevent their falling as the oxygen is under high pressure and the tanks have the potential to explode. They should be stored away from sources of heat.
- Avoid touching liquid oxygen or fill valves as liquid oxygen can burn the tissue severely. Ensure that venting is directed away from the body.
- Use only in well-ventilated areas to decrease the danger of fire.
- Maintain a distance of 6 feet or more between the source of oxygen and electrical equipment, which should be properly grounded.
- Ensure equipment is properly maintained.

Hypoxic Drive

Respirations are primarily controlled by the level of arterial carbon dioxide ($PaCO_2$) rather than the level of oxygen (PaO_2). As carbon dioxide levels rise, this normally triggers an increased rate of respiration to compensate. In some cases, such as at high altitude, respirations can be triggered by hypoxemia; this is known as hypoxic drive because the concentration of ambient oxygen is lower. This same hypoxic drive can be triggered by patients with chronic hypercarbia (≤ 70 torr). Thus, when supplementary oxygen is delivered, the hypoxic drive, which has been triggering respirations, may decrease, resulting in hypopnea or apnea. Patients who are hypoxemic may still require oxygen, but administration must be carefully managed and the patient observed for changes in respiratory rate and effort. Patients with chronic obstructive pulmonary disease receiving high fractions of inspired oxygen may actually have increased carbon dioxide levels.

Oxygen Administration

Terms related to oxygen administration include:

Flow rate (FR)	The FR is the number of liters of oxygen flow per minute. During titration, flow may be adjusted according to the patient's response, using the least amount required to obtain optimal oxygen saturation. Physicians should set the limit of allowable desaturation before polysomnography.
Fraction of inspired oxygen (FIO_2)	The FIO_2 is the percentage of oxygen in the mixture of air provided the patient. This ranges from that of room air, 21%–100%, but is usually maintained at 60% or less. FIO_2 may be expressed as a decimal or percentage: 0.50 equals 50%. When ordering oxygen for titration, the physician usually does not specify the exact FIO_2 but rather the target oxygen saturation.
Room air (RA)	RA is 21% oxygen. This is the usual air provided by positive airway pressure.

High- and Low-Flow Delivery Devices

High-flow oxygen delivery devices provide oxygen at flow rates higher than the patient's inspiratory flow rate at specific medium-to-high fraction of inspired oxygen (FIO_2), up to 100%. However a flow of 100% oxygen actually provides only 60%–80% FIO_2 to the patient because the patient also breathes in some room air, diluting the oxygen. The actual amount of oxygen received depends on the type of interface or mask. Additionally, the flow rate is actually less than the inspiratory flow rate upon actual delivery. High-flow oxygen delivery is usually not used in the sleep center. Humidification is usually required because the high flow is drying.

Low-flow oxygen delivery devices provide 100% oxygen at flow rates lower than the patient's inspiratory flow rate, but the oxygen mixes with room air, so the FIO_2 varies. Humidification is usually only required if the flow rate is 3 L/min or more. Much oxygen is wasted with exhalation, so a number of different devices to conserve oxygen are available. Interfaces include transtracheal catheters and cannulae with reservoirs.

OXYGEN INTERFACES

Oxygen interfaces are used for the delivery of oxygen to the patient.

Nasal prongs (cannulae)	This is the most common delivery system for oxygen because of ease of use, providing the fraction of inspired oxygen (FIO_2) of 24%–40% with flows at 6 L/min or less (although the maximum for infants is 2 L/min). Humidification is needed for flow rates of 4 L/min or more.
Oxygen mask	This covers the nose and mouth, delivering FIO_2 of 30%–60%, but the flow of oxygen should be maintained between 6–12 L/min to prevent rebreathing. Because of the higher flow rate, humidification should be used. Oxygen masks are usually used short-term when higher rates of oxygen are needed.
Venturi mask	Oxygen entrainment masks come with different size color-coded nozzles to control the FIO_2 accurately, with different sizes providing different FIO_2 rates, usually ranging from 24%–50%, although a FIO_2 of 35% or more is not always reliable. Flow rate is 12–15 L/min. Air-entrainment humidifiers may be used to add humidification. Oxygen entrainment masks are often used with patients who have chronic obstructive pulmonary disease.

SUPPLEMENTARY OXYGEN AND CENTRAL SLEEP APNEA

Supplementary oxygen may be used with positive airway pressure to treat central sleep apnea (CSA) not related to hypercapnia. The oxygen reduces hypoxemia, in turn, reducing reflex hyperventilation and hypocapnia to maintain the arterial carbon dioxide at an adequate level to prevent apnea in some patients. However, if the CSA is hypercapnic, oxygen therapy may cause worsening of the condition, so blood gases must be monitored. Oxygen is titrated during polysomnography until CSA resolves. In some cases, such as with heart disease, medications that improve circulation and oxygenation may relieve CSA. Others may receive stimulant medication rather than oxygen. CSA is most common in adults and premature infants. An infant with CSA is fitted with apnea alarms, which usually waken the infant and trigger respirations.

OXYGEN ADMINISTRATION DURING POLYSOMNOGRAPHY

Oxygen administration during polysomnography follows a protocol of continuous positive airway pressure (CPAP)/bilevel positive airway pressure (Bi-PAP) titration so reports are consistent. Procedures include the following:

- Ensure oxygen does not interfere with airflow sensors. Do not use two sets of nasal prongs, but rather use bifurcated dual tubes that allow for oxygen administration on one side and airflow measurements on the other; however, check to ensure that both nostrils are equal in size and patent.
- Alternately, replace the nasal pressure cannula that measures airflow with the oxygen nasal prongs, and measure directly from the oxygen tubing.

- During CPAP/Bi-PAP titration, the administration of oxygen depends on the type of interface and equipment. Check the manufacturer's guidelines for the addition of oxygen, which may be administered through an oxygen inlet nipple provided or through additional tubing and an adaptor between the humidifier and the patient.
- Keep the flow of oxygen as far away from the electrical equipment as possible.

Supplemental Low-Flow Oxygen

Supplemental low-flow oxygen is used with a polysomnogram, the use of which must be explained by the technologist. The appropriate oxygen delivery device should be in place, ensuring that the oxygen will not interfere with airflow measurements. Steps to oxygen titration include:

Initiate	Initiate low-flow supplemental oxygen at 1 L/min when oxygen saturation (SpO_2) falls below 85% on ambient room air.
Monitor	Monitor SpO_2 carefully to ensure it increases to at least 90%. Alternate monitoring methods include obtaining arterial blood gases from indwelling arterial lines and measuring transcutaneous PO_2.
Titrate	Titrate oxygen by slowly increasing the flow rate by 0.5 L/min at a time until the SpO_2 is 90% or more, but do not exceed 4 L/min without a specific physician's order. If higher levels of oxygen are needed, then different oxygen delivery devices may be indicated along with humidification.

Oxygen Troubleshooting

Oxygen troubleshooting includes the following:

- If supplemental oxygen does not increase the oxygen saturation (Sp02), this may indicate that there is a leak in the system that is interfering with oxygen delivery or that monitoring devices, such as the airflow sensor and pulse oximeter are not recording properly, so the technologist should examine these.
- The patient should be observed for mouth leaks or mouth breathing that prevents adequate intake of oxygen.
- If measurements are accurate and no problem is found with leaks, then the other equipment, such as the flowmeter and tubing should be checked for functioning and patency.
- If the Sp02 remains dangerously low, then the technologist may need to interrupt the polysomnogram and awaken the patient to ensure that a medical emergency has not occurred.
- If the patient experiences persistent low Sp02, hypoxia, and respiratory distress on awakening or is unresponsive, the technologist should contact the physician.

Pediatrics

CPAP for Obstructive Sleep Apnea

Continuous positive airway pressure (CPAP) is used for obstructive sleep apnea (OSA) in pediatric patients, which may resolve as they grow; however, some children progress to adult OSA, especially if they were not diagnosed and treated as children. Issues relevant to children include the following:

- Infants younger than 9 months may be started on CPAP immediately without prior practice or behavioral training.
- Tolerance to the interface and treatment varies widely, according to age and temperament. Many children benefit from a staged approach in which they first have polysomnography for diagnosis and are sent home with a nasal mask (hose detached) to practice wearing and adjusting to the mask before they return to the sleep center for titration.
- Fitting the mask can be challenging, and in some cases, specially molded masks to fit the child may be required. Trying a variety of interfaces may help to find one that is effective.
- Warming the tubing or using warm humidification may relieve nasal swelling and discomfort.

Titrating Continuous Positive Airway Pressure and Bilevel Positive Airway Pressure

Titrating continuous positive airway pressure (CPAP)/bilevel positive airway pressure (Bi-PAP) for pediatric patients should begin with the lowest pressure (generally 4 cm H_2O) with very slow progression because children cannot tolerate the same flow rates as adults and may develop signs of excess pressure, such as increased arousals, using accessory muscles for respiration, decrease in oxygen saturation below baseline, episodes of central apnea, and carbon dioxide retention. Manufacturer's guidelines should be followed closely. The child must be monitored continuously for signs of improvement, such as the elimination of obstructive events, decreased effort of breathing, and adequate airflow. Infants, especially those with Pierre Robin syndrome, characterized by micrognathia with a tongue that causes airflow obstruction, often have more severe obstruction during REM sleep, and the pressure needed to control symptoms during REM sleep may disturb sleep during non-REM sleep. Further, even if an infant or child is adequately titrated, requirements may change with development. Infants should be retested about every 3 months initially, extending to every year as their growth stabilizes.

Oxygen/PAP for Pulmonary Chest Disorders and Cardiac Abnormalities

Pediatric patients with pulmonary disorders (congenital or acquired abnormalities), chest wall deformities, or cardiac abnormalities may require supplementary oxygen with or without positive airway pressure. Oxygen saturation levels (baseline and during REM sleep) should be evaluated before titration to ensure that supplementary oxygen is necessary. Oxygen should be administered using the same type of supply that will be available in the home, often a concentrator, beginning with a very low flow. If the child is already receiving oxygen, this flow rate is used initially with slow increments:

- Infants: Increments of 0.25 L/min
- Children: Increments of 0.5–1 L/min

Children should be observed carefully for signs of hypoventilation related to decreased hypoxic drive (common in infants and children), so carbon dioxide must be monitored. Titration must include at least one period of REM sleep as requirements may vary from those of non-REM sleep. The age of the child and the diagnosis are important in determining how frequently the child should be reassessed.

OXYGEN/PAP FOR HYPOVENTILATION DISORDERS

Hypoventilation disorders in pediatric patients may require noninvasive ventilation (NIV)/positive airway pressure (PAP) with or without controlled respirations. Hypoventilation may relate to the following:

- Central nervous system (e.g., brain injury, Arnold-Chiari malformation): Hypoventilation is most obvious during slow-wave sleep when respirations are primarily under the control of the autonomic nervous system.
- Obstructive: This may relate to congenital malformations or obesity.
- Peripheral: Muscles of respiration cannot perform adequately.

Nocturnal hypoventilation generally occurs before onset of hypoventilation in wake time. Titration usually begins with PAP only, but humidification and volume control may be indicated for some children. Spontaneous control of respirations is titrated first, followed by a minimal synchronized intermittent mandatory ventilation rate if necessary. End expiratory pressure is increased to promote oxygenation, and the peak pressure or respiratory rate increased for carbon dioxide retention. Children with respiratory failure and progressive neuromuscular disorders may need NIV/PAP or other ventilatory support during the daytime as well as during the night.

PRIMARY RESPIRATORY FUNCTION

The primary respiratory function is to facilitate the body's cells to obtain energy from the oxidation of carbohydrates, fats, and proteins, a process that requires oxygen and generates carbon dioxide as a by-product.

Oxygen transport	Blood circulates to carry oxygen to the cells and to remove carbon dioxide by diffusion at the capillary level.
Respiration	Gas exchange occurs between the atmospheric air and the blood and between the blood and the body cell.
	The capillaries in the lungs have a lower concentration of oxygen than the alveoli, so oxygen diffuses into the blood.
	The capillaries have a higher concentration of carbon dioxide than the alveoli, so carbon dioxide diffuses into the alveoli.
Ventilation	Air flows into the lungs during inspiration and back into the atmosphere during expiration with airflow governed by variances in air pressure, airway resistance, and compliance.

VENTILATION

Ventilation carries air with oxygen into the lungs and waste products, including carbon dioxide, out of the lungs. Important factors include the following:

Air pressure variances	Inspiration: The thorax expands and lowers the pressure in the thoracic cavity relative to atmospheric pressure, drawing air into the alveoli.
	Expiration: The diaphragm relaxes, and the lungs contract; pressure inside the alveoli increases relative to atmospheric pressure, causing air to flow out of the lungs.

Airway resistance	Resistance directly relates to the size of the airway, so changes in size can increase resistance, requiring an increased effort of breathing: Bronchial contraction of smooth muscles (asthma) Mucosal hyperplasia (chronic bronchitis) Airway obstruction (tumor, mucus, foreign body) Dilation or loss of elasticity as with chronic obstructive pulmonary disease (COPD)
Compliance	The elasticity and expandability of the lungs and thoracic cavity determine the volume/pressure relationship: Compliance decreases when lung expansion is limited or "tight" (pneumothorax, pulmonary edema, atelectasis), requiring increased effort of breathing. Compliance increases with overdistention of the thorax or loss of elasticity as in COPD.

Airway resistance and compliance are issues that must be considered by the technologist when titrating for positive airway pressure because these issues along with patient effort determine the volume of airflow per inspiration.

- If compliance is decreased, which is common in obese patients or those with restrictive pulmonary disease, then higher pressure differences between inspiratory pressure and expiratory pressure are needed to ensure an adequate volume of air during ventilation.
- If compliance is increased, such as from emphysema, then lower pressure differences are needed.
- Increased airway resistance may require higher pressure to deliver an adequate volume of air.
- Increased airway resistance, such as is found in emphysema, often results in prolonged expiration, so the ratio of inspiration to expiration (I:E) may need to be adjusted from the normal 1:2 to 1:4 or more.

Hemodynamics

Hemodynamics is based on the principle that fluid flows from areas of higher pressure to areas of lower pressure:

- Systole: Pressure rises in the ventricles, closing tricuspid and mitral (atrioventricular) valves, stopping flow from the atria and preventing backflow (regurgitation). Pressure forces the pulmonic and aortic valves (semilunar valves) open, sending blood into both the aorta and pulmonary artery. Early ventricular systolic pressure is high and then falls near the end of systole as the ventricles empty, lowering the pressure in the aorta and pulmonary artery, causing atrioventricular valves to close.
- Diastole: Ventricles are relaxed and atrioventricular valves open. Pressure in the atria is lower than in the venae cavae or pulmonary veins, pulling blood into the atria with some to the ventricles. An electrical impulse is generated in the sinoatrial node, forcing the atria to contract, increasing the pressure and forcing more blood through the valves and into the ventricles. This period is atrial systole and occurs near the end of ventricular diastole.

Cardiac Output

Cardiac output is the amount of blood pumped through the ventricles during a specified period. Oxygen must be delivered to the cells to prevent tissue and organ damage, so oxygen delivery should be continuously assessed by the technologist. Normal cardiac output is about 5 L/min at rest for an adult. Under exercise or stress, this volume may multiply three or four times with concomitant changes in the heart rate (HR) and stroke volume (SV). The basic formulation for calculating cardiac output (CO) is the heart rate per minute multiplied by the stroke volume, which is the amount of blood pumped through the ventricles with each contraction. The stroke volume is controlled by preload (elasticity/volume of ventricles), afterload (systemic vascular resistance), and contractibility:

CO = HR/min X SV.

The heart rate is controlled by the autonomic nervous system. Normally, if the heart rate decreases, stroke volume increases to compensate, but with cardiomyopathies, this may not occur, so bradycardia results in a sharp decline in cardiac output.

Hemodynamic Terms

Cardiac output (CO) is the amount of blood pumped through the ventricles, usually calculated in liters per minute. Normal values at rest are 4–6 L/min.

Cardiac index (CI) is the cardiac output divided by the body surface area (BSA) [CI = CO divided by BSA]. This is essentially a measure of cardiac output tailored to the individual, based on height and weight, measured in liters per minute per square meter of body surface area. Normal values are 2.2–4.0 L/min/m^2.

Stroke volume (SV) is the amount of blood pumped through the left ventricle with each contraction, minus any blood remaining inside the ventricle at the end of systole. Normal values are 60–70 mL. The formula is below:

(CO L/min) / ((HR/min) x (1000)) = SV mL.

Pulmonary vascular resistance (PVR) is the resistance in the pulmonary arteries and arterioles against which the right ventricle has to pump during contraction. It is the mean pressure in the pulmonary vascular bed divided by blood flow. If PVR increases, SV decreases. Normal values are 1.2–3.0 units or 100–250 dynes/sec/cm^5.

Arterial Oxygen

Arterial oxygen is carried in the red blood cells by hemoglobin. Each hemoglobin molecule can carry four molecules of oxygen, with 1 g of hemoglobin equal to 1.39 mL of oxygen (100 mL arterial blood carries 0.3 mL oxygen). When the hemoglobin is fully saturated (four oxygen molecules per molecule of hemoglobin), then arterial oxygen saturation is 100%. A small amount of oxygen remains dissolved in blood (PaO_2 x 0.0031), but this has little effect on arterial oxygen content. The formula to determine arterial oxygen (CaO_2) is below:

CaO_2 = [hemoglobin x arterial oxygen saturation (SaO_2) x 1.39] + [arterial partial pressure of oxygen (PaO_2 x 0.003].

Within the sleep laboratory, a simplified formula is used to evaluate oxygen delivery (O_2D):

O2D = [stroke volume x heart rate] x SpO2.

Perfusion pressure is estimated by the systolic blood pressure:

Systolic blood pressure = cardiac output x systemic vascular resistance.

Ventilation-Perfusion

Ventilation-perfusion refers to oxygen diffusing across the alveolar membrane into the capillary blood. As oxygen in its gaseous form is exposed to the liquid blood, the oxygen dissolves until it reaches a state of equilibrium in which the partial pressure of the dissolved oxygen in the blood is equal to the partial pressure of oxygen in its gaseous state in the alveoli:

- Normal ventilation-perfusion: With normal lung function, blood passing by the alveoli is matched with an equal amount of gas, so ventilation matches perfusion (ratio 1:1).
- Low ventilation-perfusion: Shunting occurs when perfusion exceeds ventilation so that an adequate volume of blood passes by the alveoli, but the blood does not pick up adequate amounts of gas because of obstruction, such as from atelectasis.
- High ventilation-perfusion: Dead space occurs because ventilation is adequate but not blood supply so gas exchange is impaired. This can occur with pulmonary embolism and shock.
- Silent unit: No or very little exchange occurs, such as with pneumothorax or acute respiratory distress syndrome.

Oxyhemoglobin Dissociation Curve

The xyhemoglobin dissociation curve is a graph that plots the percentage of hemoglobin saturated with oxygen (y axis) and different partial pressures of oxygen (PaO_2 levels) [x axis]. A curve shift to the right represents conditions where hemoglobin has less affinity for oxygen (greater amounts of oxygen are released). A shift to the left has the opposite implications. Low pH shifts the curve to the right, enabling increased unloading of hemoglobin to tissues. Elevated oxygen shifts the curve to the left, causing increased affinity of hemoglobin for oxygen in the lungs. Small changes in fetal PO_2 result in greater loading or unloading of oxygen compared to adult hemoglobin. Because of the increased affinity for oxygen, lower tissue oxygen levels are needed to trigger unload of oxygen. Thus, the infant will have a lower PaO_2 and oxygen saturation before cyanosis is evident. Normal PaO_2 is 80–100 mm Hg, equal to 95%–98% oxygen saturation. Levels less than 40 mm Hg are dangerous.

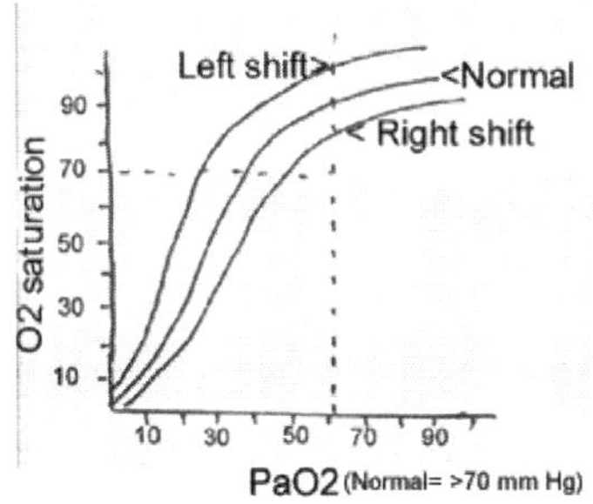

Arterial Blood Gases

Arterial blood gases are sometimes monitored to assess the effectiveness of oxygenation, ventilation, and acid-base status and to determine oxygen flow rates. Partial pressure of a gas is that exerted by each gas in a mixture of gases, proportional to its concentration, based on total atmospheric pressure of 760 mm Hg at sea level. Normal values include the following:

- Acidity/alkalinity (pH): 7.35–7.45
- Partial pressure of carbon dioxide ($PaCO_2$): 35–45 mm Hg
- Partial pressure of oxygen (PaO_2): ≥ 80 mm Hg
- Bicarbonate concentration (HCO_3): 22–26 mEq/L
- Oxygen saturation (SaO_2): ≥ 95%

The relationship between these elements, particularly the $PaCO_2$ and the PaO_2 indicates respiratory status. For example, $PaCO_2$ over 55 mm Hg and the PaO_2 under 60 mm Hg in a patient previously in good health indicates respiratory failure. There are many issues to consider. Ventilator management may require a higher $PaCO_2$ to prevent barotrauma and a lower PaO_2 to reduce oxygen toxicity.

Review Video: Blood Gases
Visit mometrix.com/academy and enter code: 611909

Hemoglobin and Hematocrit

Hemoglobin and hematocrit are particularly important in evaluating the amount of oxygen in the blood. Red blood cells (RBCs or erythrocytes) contain hemoglobin (95% of mass), which carries oxygen throughout the body. The heme portion of the cell contains iron, which binds to the oxygen.

- Hemoglobin, a protein found in erythrocytes, uses iron to bind and transport oxygen. Deficiencies of amino acids, vitamins, or minerals can cause a decrease, impacting healing and reducing oxygen to tissue. Dehydration and severe burns can cause an increase. Normal values for men are 13–18 g/dL, and for women, 12–16 g/dL.
- Hematocrit measures the percentage of packed red blood cells in 100 mL of blood. A decrease can indicate blood loss and anemia. An increase may indicate dehydration, and measurements may monitor the effects of rehydration. Normal values for men are 42%–52%, and for women, 37%–48%.

Monitoring Respirations

Monitoring respirations during polysomnography and positive airway pressure titration, entails monitoring not only actual respirations but also the intent to breathe. For example, if there is upper airway obstruction, then the airflow sensor may not register a breath, but the respiratory effort sensors (e.g., strain gauges, inductance plethysmographic devices) may indicate movement of the chest wall or the abdomen, indicating obstructive sleep apnea. If both airflow and chest wall and abdominal movement are absent, this indicates central sleep apnea. In some cases, esophageal balloon catheters can be inserted to indicate changes in thoracic volume, another indicator of the effort to breathe, which causes a negative pressure deflection. The tip of the balloon catheter must be in the lower third of the esophagus to register correct pressure changes.

Humidifiers

Humidifiers may be integrated into the positive airway pressure (PAP) device or external devices connected by tubing. When PAP therapy is delivered without humidification, the flow of pressurized air can exceed the ability of the nose to warm and moisten the air, resulting in drying of mucous membranes. The body compensates by increasing blood supply, resulting in swelling that narrows the airway and increases mouth breathing and mouth leaks. Two types of humidifiers are described below:

- Cold passover: The pressurized air passes over a reservoir of water, picking up humidity; however, warm air holds more water than cold air, so the amount of humidification is quite limited; studies show that cold-pass humidification does little to reduce the drying of mucous membranes.

- Heated: The water reservoir has a heating element, and the temperature can be adjusted up or down to control the amount of humidification. Pressurized air passes over the warmed water, picking up humidity. Heated humidification can prevent the drying of mucous membranes and relieve congestion, increasing patient comfort and compliance with treatment.

Heated Humidifiers

Heated humidifiers increase the amount of water in the pressurized air, but the level of humidification that leaves the machine and that is received by the patient can vary for a variety of reasons:

- Ambient temperature: As the air travels through the tubing, the temperature of the air changes, according to ambient temperature, so if temperature falls during the night and cools the tubing and the pressurized air, then the level of humidification also changes.
- Condensation: As air cools, its ability to hold water decreases, so condensation begins to form in the tubing, resulting in audible gurgling and decreased pressure, so preventing condensation is critically important for therapy. Solutions to reduce condensation include:
    - Increase room temperature 5 or 6 degrees at night or during cold weather.
    - Decrease the level of humidification.
    - Insulate tubing to reduce the effects of ambient temperature.
    - Use heated tubing.

Post-Study Procedures

Patient Discharge Procedures

Remove Electrodes/Sensors

Electrodes and sensors must be removed from the patient upon completion of the polysomnogram:

- If adhesive tape is used to secure electrodes or sensors, gently remove the tape while holding the skin taut, and then use adhesive remover to clean residue from the skin.
- If electrodes are attached with collodion, do not attempt to pull them loose from the skin. Soak each electrode, one at a time, with a cotton ball saturated with collodion remover or acetone to loosen the connection. As the electrode loosens, carefully remove it, and use the cotton ball to wipe any remaining collodion off the skin.
- Wipe the acetone/collodion remover off the skin with a cotton ball saturated with water or a premoistened wipe, as the chemicals can be irritating. Carefully avoid getting collodion or remover in the eyes. Ask the patient to tilt the head backward, chin up, during the procedure.
- Suggest that patients shampoo their hair as soon as possible after removal of the electroencephalogram leads because some residue may remain.

General Clean-Up

General cleanup, which is the responsibility of the sleep technologist after completion of the polysomnogram, includes the following:

- Check area to ensure patient has removed all belongings.
- Bag and label any patient belongings that remain.
- Discard all disposable items, such as tape, gauze, and nasal cannulae, in proper bags or containers.

- Empty humidifiers, and empty and clean any filters.
- Prepare reusable equipment for cleaning and disinfecting in the appropriate "dirty" service area.
- Clean and disinfect equipment, according to protocols, and return it to the proper "clean" storage area.
- Check equipment, including wires, to ensure that they are intact.
- Restock supplies as necessary.
- Return supplies and equipment to storage areas when indicated.
- Prepare the room for housekeeping, according to protocol (usually includes removing bedding).

Cleaning and Disinfecting Sensors and Interfaces

Cleaning and disinfecting sensors and interfaces must be done carefully, according to manufacturer's guidelines to prevent cross-contamination. Premoistened disinfecting wipes may be used to wipe equipment clean. Disinfectants must not be corrosive to metal or plastic.

Equipment	Disinfectant	Cleaning Procedure
Airflow sensors	Low	Wipe clean, and air dry.
Bed Linen	None	Wash and dry. Place contaminated bed linens in appropriate impermeable bag, according to facility guidelines.
Belts	Low	Soak in solution, and air dry.
Body position sensors	Low	Wipe clean, do not soak, and air dry.
Continuous positive airway pressure mask	Moderate, high grade	Soak and air dry.
Electroencephalogram electrodes	Intermediate	Wipe with acetone to remove collodion. Rinse with warm water, soak, and air dry.
Headgear	None	Wash with pure soap in warm water and dry.
Limb sensors	Low	Soak strap, and air dry. Wipe sensors clean, do not soak, and air dry.
Oximetry sensor	Low	Discard disposable adhesive, wipe clean, do not soak, and air dry.
Snap electrodes	Low	Wipe clean, do not soak, and air dry.
Snore microphone	Low	Wipe clean, do not soak, and air dry.

After Test Is Complete

When the test is completed, the technologist should turn on the lights, and tell the patient that the polysomnogram/titration is completed, usually at a predetermined time; in some cases, patients should be allowed to complete REM sleep if time allows:

- Advise the patient that calibrations need to be repeated to ensure that the equipment has been functioning properly. If doing a positive airway pressure titration, remove the patients mask before shutting off the machine.
- Allow the patient to use the bathroom, if necessary.
- Repeat the equipment calibrations and biocalibrations in the same manner as done before the test, documenting any discrepancies or indications of malfunctions.
- Remove all electrodes and sensors.

- Follow the manufacturer's instructions in terminating the recording.
- Assist the patient as necessary for transfer (if an inpatient) or to dress and prepare to leave. In some cases, shower facilities are available for patients.
- Provide a morning questionnaire for the patient to fill out.
- Assist patient to the exit.

AMA Form

Complete an Against Medical Advice (AMA) form if the patient insists on ending the polysomnogram (PSG) prematurely. An over-night nocturnal PSG should last for 6 hours or more to obtain adequate data, and a split-night PSG should have time for 3 hours of titration. Noting the exact time that the PSG begins and ends is necessary. Because Medicare and other insurance may not pay for an incomplete procedure, any interruption should be noted, such as an emergency that necessitates early termination. The procedure to complete an AMA typically includes the following:

- Evaluate and document the patient's level of comprehension and competence to make decisions.
- Explain why the test should not be terminated early, such as the need for 6 hours of recording. Consequences, such as inadequate data and denial of payment by Medicare or other insurance carriers.
- Suggest alternatives, such as a short break or a walk in the facility.
- Explore reasons, such as anxiety, fear, or discomfort.
- If unable to convince the patient to continue and the patient is competent, ask the patient to sign the AMA form; ensure that the patient has transportation available.
- If patient is confused or deemed incompetent to make a decision because of drugs, alcohol, or other physical condition, then do not allow the patient to leave. Call security, family members, or caregivers as necessary.

Morning Questionnaire

Morning questionnaires are completed when the polysomnogram (PSG) is terminated because the sleep experience in the sleep center may be profoundly different from that normally experienced by the patient. The questionnaire is relatively short as patients may want to leave, especially if they have to go to work. Typical questions include the patient's perceptions about the following:

- Sleep quality
- Onset to sleep time
- Number of arousals
- Total sleep time.
- Differences between home sleep and lab sleep
- Sleepiness on awakening

The questionnaire may take the form of a simple checklist, or the technologist may ask specific questions. However, if the questionnaire is in paper form, the technologist should always review the answers before the patient leaves the facility and ask for clarification if more information is needed. If, for example, the patient reports that sleep was very different from usual, a repeat PSG may be indicated.

Patient Follow-Up

Patient follow-up is almost always necessary to ensure compliance with positive airway pressure. Patients may be nervous and confused when they first receive instructions, so simply sending the patient home with equipment after titration may not be adequate. The type of follow-up and the responsibility varies with sleep centers but is often part of the sleep technologist's job description and should include the following:

Contact	Make contact usually at 2 days, 1 week, 2 weeks, 6 weeks, 6 months, and yearly by telephone or e-mail.The patient's use of positive airway pressure equipment, including frequency and duration to determine compliance.Interface or equipment problems, daytime sleepiness, and snoring.
Education	Within the first month of therapy: Suggest classes or instruction regarding the patient's sleep disorder and appropriate treatments. Give patients contact information in case they have questions.
Support	The technologist can keep in touch with the patient about the following: A.W.A.K.E. Ongoing peer support groups (often supervised or led by the technologist)

Follow-Up Education

Follow-up education is an important component of treating sleep disorders, so classes should be offered in a variety of settings and at different times to accommodate those with work or family. Educational content should include the following information:

- Disorders: Characteristics of different diagnoses and implications for health
- Treatment: Positive airway pressure (PAP), bilevel positive airway pressure, and automatic positive airway pressure
- Medicare or other Insurance: Coverage, limitations, and requirements
- Adverse effects: Nasal congestion, mouth leaks, skin irritations, and methods of dealing with them
- Travel: Transporting and using PAP outside of the home
- Resources: Classes, Internet, and books
- Equipment: Use, storage, cleaning, and parts replacement
- Safety: General issues, including protection of wiring and use of oxygen
- Partner problems: Issues related to partner complaints and intimacy; Desensitization techniques
- Sleep hygiene: Basic techniques for sleeping
- Symptoms: Snoring, sleepiness, and arousals
- Humidification: Purpose, use, and troubleshooting

ASAA's A.W.A.K.E. Program

The America Sleep Apnea Association's (ASAA's) A.W.A.K.E. (Alert, Well, And Keeping Energetic) program is comprised of self-help groups. A coordinator leads the meetings, and members often invite guest speakers to discuss topics of interest to the group. Meetings are available in all 50 states but may not be readily available in rural areas. Coordinators are often sleep professionals, although this is not a requirement. Groups are advised, however, to be sponsored by a sleep professional who can serve as a resource for the group. The ASAA provides guidelines for those wanting to establish A.W.A.K.E. groups. The goal of A.W.A.K.E. is to educate people about sleep apnea so that people are able to manage their health and to provide guidance and ongoing support. ASAA provides suggested topics for meetings, and meeting frequency varies from monthly to quarterly. ASAA also provides educational materials, such as reports, newsletters, and videos. Members of A.W.A.K.E. are not required to join ASAA.

FOSQ

The Functional Outcomes of Sleep Questionnaire (FOSQ), developed by T. E. Weaver, is an effective tool to assess whether excessive sleepiness persists. Patients should be assessed with FOSQ for improvement after completing the polysomnogram and positive airway pressure titration. The patients respond to fourteen questions about activities with the following rating scale:

0 = Do not do this.
1 = Strongly yes
2 = Moderately yes
3 = Slightly yes.
4 = No

The questions relate to being sleepy or tired and the ability to concentrate, remember things, eat, do hobbies, work about the home, operate motor vehicles, manage financial affairs, volunteer, talk on the phone, and visit with family or friends. Other questions relate to the person's ability to enjoy a number of activities, such as watching television or going to concerts or being as active as they would like to be or expect to be for their age. The last questions relate to the impact being tired and sleepy has on arousal and sexual activity.

Berlin Questionnaire

The Berlin Questionnaire (1996) is most often used for screening those at risk for obstructive sleep apnea, but it is also occasionally used to determine progress after the onset of treatment with positive airway pressure. It comprises a total of fourteen questions in three categories, although height and weight are also important for calculating the body mass index (BMI):

- Category 1 (snoring): Presence, characteristics, frequency, impact on bed partner/others, and episodes of apnea
- Category 2 (daytime tiredness or fatigue): Presence, frequency, and occurrences while driving (falling asleep)
- Category 3 (hypertension): Positive if hypertension present or BMI is 30 kg/m^2 or more

Patients are classified as high or low risk based on positive findings in the different categories. High risk means that positive scores are found in two or three categories. Low risk means that positive scores are found in one category or fewer.

Cleaning and Care of Equipment

Cleaning and care of equipment is very important so before beginning home treatment with positive airway pressure, patients need to be instructed on how to do this properly.

Daily maintenance	Clean the mask daily with soapy water, rinse with water or white vinegar, and air dry to prevent skin irritation or infection.
	Rinse tubing with water or a white vinegar mixture, and hang to dry so that any fluid drains to prevent mold from growing inside the tubing.
Monthly maintenance	Remove and clean disposable filter (usually in the back of the machine) with soapy water, rinse thoroughly, and air dry before reuse.
	Replace paper filters. Filters may need to be replaced more frequently in a dusty, dirty environment or one with animal hair.
Humidifier care	Always empty the reservoir each day.
	Wash the reservoir in warm, soapy water, rinse thoroughly with water or a vinegar solution, and air dry.

	Use only distilled water for humidification.

Travel Considerations for PAP Use

Travel considerations for patients using positive airway pressure (PAP), must be discussed as patients frequently need to travel; they should be advised to always carry their PAP equipment with them as symptoms may return after missing even 1 day of treatment.

Transporting equipment	Secure in a carrying case (usually provided).
	If traveling by plane, carry the equipment, and store in the passenger compartment as rough handling or temperature extremes in the luggage storage area may damage equipment.
Power issues	Take voltage convertors and adaptors as needed if traveling overseas.
	Take a power extension cord.
	Provide battery-powered backup if necessary (e.g., for camping).
Humidifier	Carry distilled water, or purchase on arrival.
	Compensate for lack of a humidifier with a saline nasal spray or water-soluble gel.
Altitude adjustments	Check altitude and manufacturer's guidelines for adjusting pressure.

HIPAA

The Health Insurance Portability and Accountability Act (HIPAA) addresses the rights of the individual related to privacy of health information. The technologist must not release any information or documentation about a patient's condition or treatment without consent, as the individual has the right to determine who has access to personal information. Personal information about the patient is considered protected health information and consists of any identifying or personal information about the patient, such as health history, condition, treatments in any form, and any documentation, including electronic, verbal, or written. Personal information can be shared with parents of minors, spouses, legal guardians, those with durable power of attorney for the patient, and those involved in the care of the patient, such as physicians, without a specific release, but the patient should always be consulted if personal information is to be discussed with others present to ensure there is no objection. Failure to comply with HIPAA regulations can make a technologist liable for legal action.

Confidentiality

Confidentiality is the obligation that is present in a professional–patient relationship. Technologists are under an obligation to protect the information they possess concerning the patient and family. Care should be taken to safeguard that information and provide the privacy that the family deserves. This is accomplished through the use of required passwords when the family calls for information about the patient and through the limitations of who is allowed to visit. There may be times when confidentiality must be broken to save the life of a patient, but those circumstances are rare. The technologist must make all efforts to safeguard patient records and identification. Computerized record-keeping should be done in such a way that the screen is not visible to others, and paper records must be secured.

PATIENTS' RIGHTS

Patients' (families') rights concerning what to expect from a health care organization are outlined in the standards of both the Joint Commission and the National Committee for Quality Assurance. Rights include:

- Respect for the patient, including personal dignity and psychosocial, spiritual, and cultural considerations
- Response to needs related to access and pain control
- Ability to make decisions about care, including informed consent, advance directives, and end-of-life care
- Procedure for registering complaints or grievances
- Protection of confidentiality and privacy
- Freedom from abuse or neglect
- Protection during research and information related to ethical issues of research
- Appraisal of outcomes, including unexpected outcomes
- Information about organization, services, and practitioners
- Appeal procedures for decisions regarding benefits and quality of care
- Organizational code of ethical behavior
- Procedures for donating and procuring organs and tissue

SUMMARIZING AND STORING DATA

DATA SUMMARY

A data summary must be completed once the polysomnogram is completed and should include the following:

- Times: Lights on and lights off
- Sleep: Overall quality of sleep and unusual sleep behavior
- Snoring: Presence, frequency, duration, and type
- Oxygen saturation (SpO_2): Lowest SpO_2 recorded and duration
- Abnormal electroencephalogram findings: Presence, frequency, duration, and type
- Periodic leg movements in sleep: Presence, frequency, and severity
- Body positions: Positions, time of changing positions, and effects of change on vital signs, respirations, sleep quality, and snoring
- Respiratory abnormalities: Type of disturbance, frequency, duration, and associations (e.g., position changes)
- Continuous positive airway pressure (CPAP) titration: If included, optimal setting to relieve symptoms and any difficulties or abnormalities related to CPAP

DATA

Data should be saved, stored, and properly identified, according to manufacturer's guidelines and protocol, upon completion of the polysomnogram (PSG). Data may be stored in analog or digital form, depending on the equipment, but protocols must be followed carefully to ensure patient confidentiality and integrity of the recordings. The PSG is usually videotaped so that the evaluator can view patient activity while studying the recordings. The technologist should begin the videotaping when applying the sensors, and this recording should be maintained for legal reasons as well in case the patient reports inappropriate behavior or contact, especially since the sleep technologist is often the only other person present. Some older equipment may save videos in a video home system format for viewing on a videocassette recorder, but most newer equipment is digital. Digital videos are easily stored electronically and can be viewed onscreen while simultaneously evaluating the recordings.

CQI

Continuous Quality Improvement (CQI) emphasizes the organization and systems and processes within that organization rather than individuals. It recognizes internal customers (staff) and external customers (patients) and uses data to improve processes. CQI represents the concept that most processes can be improved. CQI uses the scientific method of experimentation to meet needs and improve services and uses various tools, such as brainstorming, multivoting, various charts and diagrams, storyboarding, and meetings. Core concepts include the following:

- Quality and success are meeting or exceeding internal and external customer's needs and expectations.
- Problems related to processes and variations in process lead to variations in results.
- Changes can be made in small steps.

Steps to CQI include the following:

- Forming a knowledgeable team
- Identifying and defining measures used to determine success
- Brainstorming strategies for change
- Plan, collect, and use data as part of making decisions
- Test changes and revise or refine as needed

PDCA

Plan-Do-Check-Act (PDCA) or the Shewhart cycle is a method of continuous quality assurance. PDCA is simple and understandable; however, it may be difficult to maintain this cycle consistently because of a lack of focus and commitment. PDCA may be more suited to solving specific problems than organization-wide problems:

- Plan: Planning encompasses identifying, analyzing and defining the problem, setting goals, and establishing a process that coordinates with leadership. Extensive brainstorming, including fishbone diagrams, identifies problematic processes and lists current process steps. Data are collected and analyzed, and root-cause analysis is completed.
- Do: Doing involves generating solutions from which to select one or more and then implementing the solution on a trial basis.
- Check: Checking involves gathering and analyzing data to determine the effectiveness of the solution. If effective, then continue to Act; if not, return to Plan and pick a different solution. (Study may replace Check; that is, PDSA.)
- Act: Act entails identifying changes that need to be done to implement solutions fully, adopting solutions, and continuing to monitor results while picking another improvement project.

Sleep Center Staff

Sleep center staff must include a Medical Director with a license to practice, who must be a diplomate of the American Board of Sleep Medicine (ABSM) or someone who has been accepted by the ABSM to take the certification exam. The job description for staff positions should be detailed, clear, and updated yearly. Staff positions may include a clerical coordinator, polysomnographic technologist, polysomnographic technician, and polysomnographic trainee. The number of staff required depends on the size and patient volume of the center. Staffing includes both daytime and nighttime hours. Centers vary in the shift duration: five 8-hour shifts, four 10-hour shifts, or three 12-hour shifts, but overtime pay may be a consideration with longer shifts. The formula for calculating full-time equivalent (FTE) staffing helps to determine staffing needs:

- 40 hr/wk x 52 wk/yr = 1 FTE.
- 20 hr/wk x 52 wk/yr = 0.5 FTE.

Staffing must include coverage and policies for breaks and meals.

Productivity Monitoring

Productivity monitoring assesses the efficiency of the sleep center and is based on the evaluation of the full-time equivalent staff and patient volume. Units of service (UOS) are the number of patients in a period of time (e.g., a pay period, which may be weekly, biweekly, or monthly). The formula for calculating productivity is shown below:

Total hours worked/UOS (number of patients) = hours/patient.

It may be more accurate to include the average cancellation rate and subtract that from the UOS. For example, if 20 patients are typically scheduled in one week but 10% usually cancel, then determine UOS with the following:

$$20 \times .10 = 2$$

$$20 - 2 = 18 \text{ (adjusted UOS)}$$

Productivity monitoring must be done on an ongoing basis as staffing may need to be adjusted if the sleep center patient census decreases or increases.

Record Scoring

Scoring of the Polysomnogram

Correct scoring of the polysomnogram depends in part on quality assurance efforts. Each epoch must be scored for the stage of sleep, arousals, respiratory events, and limb movements. Computerized scoring may be used but must be quality-controlled and verified. Interscorer reliability testing must be completed with a certified sleep specialist serving as the reference scorer. Interscorer reliability scoring must be done on 200 consecutive epochs (30 seconds) for three or more patients quarterly. There must be agreement in all scoring areas between the reference scorer and other scorers. Every study must include a complete epoch-by-epoch study of all raw data, and the sleep technologist must sign to signify that a complete review of the data was completed. The signed form may be kept as part of the patient's record or separately. Interscorer reliability scoring must be done on four portable monitoring recordings (200 epochs for constant analysis of 30–180 seconds) each year for labs that use portable recording devices outside of the facility.

Staging Sleep and Arousal

Neurotransmitters Involved in Sleep

Neurotransmitters involved in sleep include the following:

Acetylcholine	Levels increase during the wake state and during REM sleep, but levels decrease during stages 1, 2, and 3 non-REM sleep.
Adenosine	Levels increase during periods of sleep deprivation and decrease when sleeping to recover. Some drugs, such as theophylline and caffeine, suppress the function of adenosine.
Dopamine	Levels increase during the wake state and during REM sleep. Some stimulants, such as methamphetamine, increase levels.
Gamma-aminobutyric acid	Levels increase to inhibit the central nervous system.
Glutamate	Levels increase to stimulate the central nervous system.
Glycine	Levels increase to inhibit the motor nervous system at the spinal cord to cause atonia during REM sleep.
Histamine	Levels increase during the wake state. Agents that block histamine-1 receptors increase drowsiness.
Hypocretin 1, 2	Levels increase during the wake state and regulate the circadian cycle. Impairment of hypocretin production or utilization can cause narcolepsy.
Immunomodulators with sleep factors	Levels increase non-REM sleep (insulin, interleukin I, interferon-α_2, tumor necrosis factor).
	Levels increase REM sleep (somatostatin, growth hormone, prolactin).
	Levels increase both non-REM and REM sleep (prostaglandin D2, growth hormone–releasing factor).
	Levels inhibit sleep (glucocorticoids, prostaglandin E2, corticotropin-releasing factor, thyrotropin-releasing hormone).

Melatonin	Levels increase during the evening and night and begin to decrease in the morning, helping to control the sleep–wake cycle.
Norepinephrine	Levels increase to maintain the awake state, so levels decrease during stages 1, 2, and 3 non-REM sleep and are absent in REM sleep.
Serotonin	Levels increase during the awake state but decrease during non-REM and REM sleep to help regulate sleep onset with lowest levels during REM.

RETICULAR FORMATION

The reticular formation, located in the brainstem, receives neural impulses from everywhere in the body and is connected to both the cerebellum, which controls movement, balance, and coordination, and the limbic system (deep brain structures).

- The ascending pathways (dorsal and ventral), referred to as the reticular activating system (RAS), carry sensory information to the forebrain and cerebral cortex, and use a feedback method to control sleep and awake states. Sensory input and activity in the RAS bring about arousal and maintain the awake state. The RAS is linked to the motor system and controls movement during the awake state and atonia during REM sleep.
- The descending reticular formation receives input from the hypothalamus and is involved in activation of the autonomic nervous system.

LIMBIC SYSTEM

The limbic system, in the region of the diencephalon, is essential to regulation of emotion, hormones, mood, and pain or pleasure sensations. The limbic system is comprised of several structures, including:

- Amygdala: This is an almond-shaped grouping of nuclei that are responsible for mediating arousal, emotion, and fear responses, as well as hormones.
- Cingulate gyrus: This structure is responsible for matching sensory input with emotional response.
- Hippocampus: This is a group of neurons responsible for organizing and processing memories, spatial relationships, and emotional regulation.
- Hypothalamus: This is a structure that is involved in almost all body processes, to include autonomic functions, emotions, homeostasis, endocrine processes, and sleep regulation.
- Thalamus: This is a group of cells that mediates motor function, and receives, processes, and relays sensory signals to and from the cortex, playing an important role in sleep. Fibers release neurotransmitters that help to control arousal.

DIENCEPHALON

The diencephalon is located above the brainstem and between the cerebral hemispheres. It comprises primarily gray matter and surrounds the third ventricle. The diencephalon contains a number of structures important to sleep and arousal.

- Thalamus: This gland receives sensory input from other parts of the central nervous system and carries them to appropriate areas of the cerebral cortex. The thalamus serves as a gateway and also an editor for sensory input (except for smell).

- Hypothalamus: This gland regulates heart rate, blood pressure, temperature, fluid and electrolyte balance, hunger, weight, stomach, intestines, and sleep; and produces substances that stimulate the pituitary gland to release hormones.
- Optic chiasm: The optic nerves cross in this area anterior to the pituitary gland.
- Posterior pituitary gland: This gland stores and secretes oxytocin and antidiuretic hormone, which are produced by the hypothalamus.
- Mamillary bodies: These are active in the memory of smells.
- Pineal gland: This gland is attached to the third ventricle; it produces melatonin and mediates sleep.

WAKEFULNESS

Wakefulness (stage W) can be characterized by an electroencephalogram (EEG), an electromyogram (EMG), and an electrooculogram (EOG). Scoring is done by epochs, generally a 30-second record (300 mm), with only one stage of sleep scored for each epoch even though the sleep stage may vary. The epoch is assigned the primary sleep stage.

EEG	Varies according to level of wakefulness: Awake/alert (eyes open): There is low-voltage and high-frequency activity. Relaxed: There is low-frequency activity. Sleepy (eyes closed): Alpha activity (8–13 cycles/sec) is more than 50% of epoch and is observed most often from the occipital leads but may be present in the central leads or the EOG channel; alpha activity abates if the eyes are open.
EMG	There is various motor activity on the anterior tibial EMG with high-voltage activity on the chin EMG.
EOG	Varies according to level of wakefulness: Awake/alert: There is frequent blinking and rapid eye movements. Sleepy (eyes closed): Movements are slow and rolling, preceding stage 1 non REM sleep.

SCORING

Stage W (wakefulness) may vary from wide awake and alert to drowsy; alpha rhythms are usually present if the patient's eyes are closed, although about 10% of patients do not exhibit alpha rhythms.

An epoch is scored stage W with these findings:

- About 50% or more of epoch demonstrates alpha rhythm (occipital leads).
- Eye blinks occur with a frequency of 0.5–2 Hz or reading eye movements (slow phase in one direction and rapid phase in the other), or irregular conjugate REMs occur with normal or increased chin electromyogram activity (usually amplitude is higher than during stages of sleep).

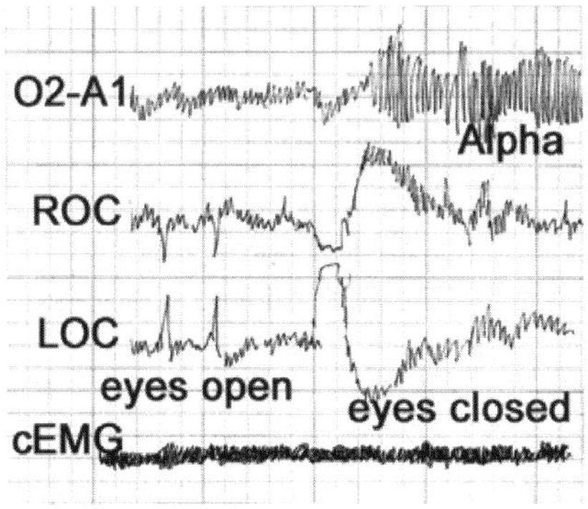

Stage 1 Non-REM Sleep

Stage 1 non-REM sleep is the transitional period between wakefulness and sleep and may occur with initial onset of sleep or after arousal. In adults, stage 1 non-REM sleep occurs in 2%–5% of total sleep time. This stage usually lasts only a few minutes before the patient enters stage 2 non-REM sleep. The patient is easily aroused in stage 1. Stage 1 non-REM sleep is characterized on the electroencephalogram (EEG), electromyogram (EMG), and electrooculogram (EOG) as follows:

EEG	Alpha activity ceases or decreases to less than 50% of epoch.
	Activity is low amplitude and mixed frequency (2–7 Hz).
	Vertex sharp negative waves (V waves) are over the central scalp area.
	Children and adolescents have high-voltage synchronous bursts of theta activity.
	No sleep spindles or K complexes or 3 minutes or more between episodes are seen.
EMG	High-voltage activity in a chin EMG is similar to or less than during stage W.
EOG	There are no REMs.
	There is some evidence of slow-rolling eye movement, especially at onset, with initial deflection of more than 500 milliseconds.

Scoring

Scoring stage 1 non-REM sleep includes alpha waves that attenuate (but only if stage W included alpha waves), and low-amplitude, mixed-frequency activity that occurs for more than 50% of epoch. Stage 1 non-REM sleep is generally characterized by slow eye movements, V waves, and low-amplitude, mixed-frequency electroencephalogram (EEG) activity. If stage W does not include alpha waves, then stage 1 non-REM sleep is scored with one or more of the following:

- Slowing of EEG background frequencies by 1 Hz or more from stage W with activity ranging from 4–7 Hz
- V waves
- Slow eye movements

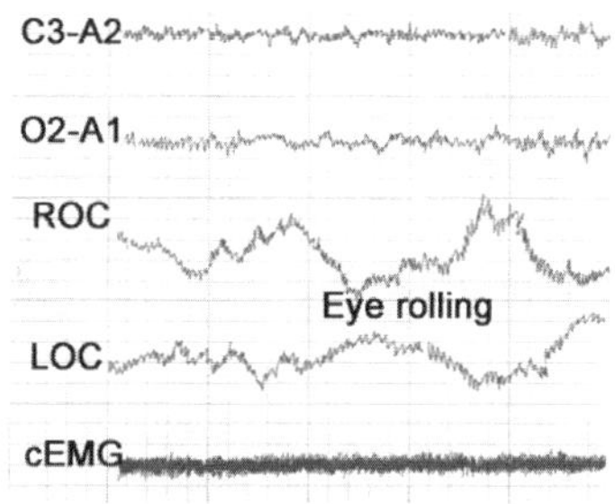

Stage 2 Non-REM Sleep

Stage 2 non-REM sleep occupies about 45%–55% of total sleep time for adults. Stage 2 non-REM sleep is characterized on electroencephalogram (EEG), electromyogram (EMG), and electrooculogram (EOG) as described below:

EEG	Activity is low voltage, mixed frequency.
	K complexes (sharp negative wave preceding slower positive wave, persisting > 0.5 seconds) and sleep spindles (bursts of rhythmic activity 12–15 Hz, persisting for □ 0.5 seconds) are evident but may not appear in each epoch. Stage 2 is characterized by intervening periods between K complexes or sleep spindles of less than 3 minutes, unrelated to arousal. Normal K-complex activity is 1–3/min in young adults.
	Delta activity is less than 20% of epoch.
	Abrupt K-complex clusters and delta waves may indicate arousal.
EMG	Low-voltage muscle activity is shown on a chin EMG.
EOG	Occasional slow-rolling eye movements are observed at onset, but more commonly, there is an absence of movement.

Scoring

Scoring stage 2 non-REM sleep must take into consideration both K complexes and sleep spindles, which characterize this stage of sleep.

- Beginning: The appearance of one or more K complexes (not associated with arousal) and one or more sleep spindles signals the beginning.
- Continuing: The electroencephalogram (EEG) shows low-amplitude, mixed-frequency activity. Epoch remains stage 2 non-REM even without K complexes or sleep spindles if the activity was preceded by a K complex (not associated with arousal) or sleep spindle.

- Termination: The end occurs with transition to another stage of sleep, arousal (reverts to stage 1 non-REM until the recurrence of a K complex without arousal or sleep spindle), or major body movement with slow eye movements on electrooculogram and low-amplitude, high-frequency EEG activity.

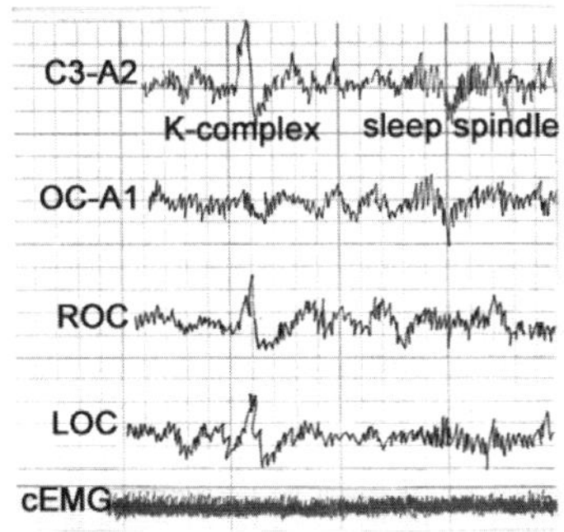

Stage 3 Non-REM Sleep

Stage 3 non-REM sleep (formerly stages 3 and 4), also referred to as slow-wave sleep (SWS) or delta sleep, accounts for about 20% of total sleep time for adults. This percentage and amplitude of delta activity is higher for adolescents and lower for older adults. Stage 3 occurs during the first half of sleep. The patient is not easily aroused from stage 3 sleep by external stimuli, such as noise or movement. Parasomnias (e.g., sleep walking, enuresis, night terrors) occur during this stage. Stage 3 non-REM sleep is characterized on electroencephalogram (EEG), electromyogram (EMG), and electrooculogram (EOG) as described below:

EEG	Delta activity (> 75 microvolts lasting ≥ 0.5 seconds, 0.5–2 Hz) is evident for 20%–50% or more of epoch.
	Sleep spindles may occur.
EMG	There is lower voltage activity in the chin EMG than in stages 1 or 2.
EOG	There is usually no activity.

Scoring

Scoring stage 3 non-REM sleep, also referred to as slow-wave or delta sleep, begins when delta waves occur in 20% or more of an epoch. These slow waves are typically reflected in the electrooculogram channels although eye movements do not usually occur with stage 3 non-REM sleep. Sleep spindles may occur at times. Slow-wave activity is in the frequency of 0.5–2 Hz with an amplitude of 0.75 microvolts (frontal) and a duration of 0.5 seconds or more. The chin electromyogram usually shows lower amplitude than in stage 2 non-REM sleep. With the previous staging that divided stage 3 into stages 3 and 4, stage 3 was scored when delta waves occurred in 20%–50% of an epoch, and stage 4, when they occurred in 50% or more of an epoch.

REM Sleep

REM sleep has both a tonic stage that occurs without eye movement and a phasic stage with REMs; it occupies about 25% of total sleep time for adults. Dreaming most often occurs during REM sleep as well as sexual arousal (penile/clitoral erection). The electrocardiogram may show variations in heart rate, and sensors may indicate differences in respirations related to the phasic stage. Nightmares and REM sleep behavior disorder occur during REM sleep. Patients arouse less easily from REM sleep. Non-REM and REM cycles typically occur about every 1.5–2 hours.

Electroencephalogram	Low-voltage, mixed-frequency activity with sawtooth theta waves is often evident.

	Sleep spindles and K complexes are absent.
Electromyogram	Usually there is no activity because of atonia associated with REM sleep, although bursts of activity may occur during the phasic stage.
Electrooculogram	There are bursts of rapid conjugate movements during the phasic stage.

Scoring

Scoring REM sleep begins with rapid eye movements (REM) [< 500 milliseconds], which are often preceded by sawtooth waves on the electroencephalogram (EEG) [2–6 Hz]. Because of the atonia associated with REM sleep, electromyogram (EMG) activity is low although brief bursts of activity (< 0.25 seconds) may occur. Onset: The EEG shows low amplitude with mixed frequency and a low tone on the chin EMG (cEMG). Continuation: With or without REM, following one or more episodes of REM, the cEMG continues to show low tone, the EEG remains unchanged, and there is no evidence of K complexes or sleep spindles. Termination: One of following occurs: (1) transition to stage W or stage 3 non-REM; (2) an increase in cEMG tone and criteria for stage 1 non-REM are met; (3) arousal occurs followed by stage 1 non-REM findings (mixed-frequency EEG and slow eye movement); (4) major body movement is followed by slow eye movement and a low amplitude EEG with mixed frequency and no K complexes or sleep spindles (stage 1 non-REM); and (5) one or more non-arousal-associated K complexes or sleep spindles in the first half of epoch without REM.

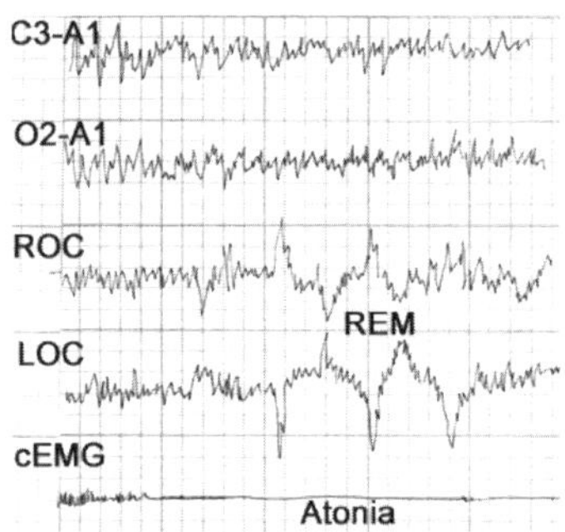

Transition Period Between Stage 2 Non-REM and REM

The transition period between stage 2 non-REM and REM is scored, according to the following guidelines:

- Score REM if there is a drop in chin electromyogram (cEMG) tone similar to that found in REM in the first half of epoch even without REM with the absence of non-arousal-associated K complexes and sleep spindles.
- Score REM if there are minimal cEMG tones (but no drop) and the absence of non-arousal-associated K complexes and sleep spindles even without REM.
- Score stage 2 non-REM if there is a drop in cEMG to REM but the presence of non-arousal-associated K complexes or sleep spindles and the absence of REM.

Major Body Movements

Major body movements may cause movement and muscle artifacts that obscure readings, sometimes making it impossible to determine the stage of sleep for that particular epoch. An epoch that follows sleep in which 50% or more is obscured by movement is considered movement time. Epochs that include major body movements are scored with the following criteria:

- Score as stage W if alpha rhythm is present for some part of the epoch.
- Score as stage W without alpha rhythm if the major body movement is preceded or followed by stage W.

If the first two criteria do not apply, score the epoch the same as the epoch that follows the major body movement.

Arousals

Arousals are brief sleep disturbances, persisting less than an epoch but interrupting sleep continuity. Arousals indicate fragmented sleep and are associated with daytime drowsiness. Arousals tend to occur more frequently with age. Arousals should be scored, using information from both occipital and central leads. Additional information can be gleaned by observing other electroencephalogram (EEG) channels and respiratory events, but these findings do not alter the basic scoring rules.

- Score arousal for all stages if after 10 or more seconds of sleep, there is a sudden change in EEG frequency, including alpha, theta, or frequencies of 16 Hz or more without spindles, persisting for at least 3 seconds.
- During REM sleep, score arousal if there is an increase in the chin electromyogram at the same time, persisting for 1 second or more.

Pediatric Sleep Scoring

Pediatric sleep scoring rules apply to children 2 months post-term or older. Because of variations in developmental sleep patterns in pediatric patients, sleep is scored with one additional stage (non-REM). Some findings are age-related.

- Sleep spindles occur at 2–3 months or older.
- K complexes and slow-wave activity (≥ 75 microvolts, 0.5–2 Hz) occur at 4–6 months or older.
- Sleep stages 1, 2, and 3 non-REM can be scored in most infants at 5–6 months or older.
- Non-electroencephalographic events can help differentiate non-REM from REM sleep in infants 6 months or younger.
    - REM: chin electromyogram (cEMG) atonia, irregular respirations, REM, and transient muscle activity
    - Non-REM: cEMG tone, regular respirations, and no or rare vertical eye movements

Non-REM Sleep Scoring

Pediatric non-REM sleep scoring depends on the age of the infant or child. Criteria for staging non-REM include the following:

Findings	Scoring
No sleep spindles, K complexes, or high-amplitude, slow-wave activity (0.5–2 Hz) are present in any epoch.	Score as non-REM.

Findings	Scoring
Some epochs contain sleep spindles or K complexes, but the remaining epochs have no slow-wave activity for 20% or more of epochs.	Score as stage 2 non-REM for epochs with sleep spindles or K complexes and non-REM for the rest.
Some epochs contain 20% or more slow-wave activity (score as stage 3 non-REM), but there are no K complexes or sleep spindles in the remaining epochs.	Score as stage 3 non-REM for epochs with slow-wave activity and non-REM for the rest.
Some epochs contain sleep spindles or K complexes, and slow-wave activity occurs in other epochs.	Do not score as non-REM, but score as stage 1, 2, or 3 non-REM, according to guidelines for older children and adults.

DPR

The dominant posterior rhythm (DPR) in pediatric patients (infants) is slower over occipital derivations. Electroencephalographic (EEG) readings for infants and children vary, according to age and stage of development.

Age	Findings (Occipital)
3–4 months or younger	Slow, irregular potential changes only
3–4 months (75%)	Irregular amplitude of 50–100 microvolts and a frequency of 3.5–4.5 Hz; attenuates/blocks with eye opening; occurs with passive eye closing
5–6 months up to 12 months (70%)	Amplitude of 50–110 microvolts; a frequency 5–6 Hz
3 years (82%)	Mean frequency of 8 Hz or more (7.5–9.5 Hz)
9 years (65%)	Average amplitude of 50–60 microvolts; mean frequency of 9 Hz; between 6–9 years, 9% with amplitude of 100 microvolts; alpha activity of 30 microvolts or less, rare in children.
15 years (65%)	Mean frequency of 10 Hz
Adults	Amplitude of 50 microvolts or less; a frequency of 8.5-13 Hz; reactive to eye opening

Stage W

Pediatric scoring of stage W uses the dominant posterior rhythm (DPR) rather than the term alpha rhythm when scoring stage W and stages non-REM, using the following criteria:

- Stage W: When 50% or more of epoch has reactive alpha waves or age- appropriate DPR, score stage W.
- Stage W: If there is no reactive alpha waves or age-appropriate DPR, score W with:
  - Eye blinks (vertical eye movements) with a frequency 0.5–2 Hz. Occipital sharp waves occur 100–500 milliseconds after eye blinks and are monophasic or biphasic, 200 microvolts or less, and usually last 200–400 milliseconds.
  - Reading eye movements (e.g., with reading or scanning environment) of a usual duration of 150–250 milliseconds with an amplitude 65 microvolts or less.
  - Irregular conjugate REM and a normal or increased chin electromyogram tone. REM may occur while the child is awake if scanning the environment.
  - Spontaneous eye closure, which indicates drowsiness (infant).

STAGES NON-REM AND REM

Pediatric scoring for stages 1, 2, and 3 non-REM and REM is as follows:

Stage 1 non-REM	With dominant posterior rhythm (DPR), if DPR is attenuated or replaced for more than half of the epoch by low-amplitude, mixed-frequency activity, score as stage 1 non-REM. Without DPR, score with any of the following: Slowing of 1–2 Hz or more from stage W and activity in 4–7 Hz range Slow eye movements Vertex sharp waves Rhythmic anterior theta activity Hypnagogic hypersynchrony High-amplitude, rhythmic 3–5 Hz activity (diffuse to occipital)
Stage 2 non-REM	Score as in adults. Sleep spindles usually occur in infants by 4–6 weeks, and K complexes, by 5–6 months.
Stage 3 non-REM	Score as in adults. Slow-wave activity often ranges from 100–400 microvolt's in children.
REM	Score as in adults. Activity resembles adults, but frequency increases with age from 3 Hz at 7 weeks, 4–5 Hz (sawtooth) at 5 months, 4–6 Hz at 9 months, and 5–7 Hz (runs and notched thetas) at 1–5 years.

Scoring Respiratory Events

SCORING APNEAS

Scoring apneas involves scoring from the nadir of the preceding breath to the beginning of the next normal breath, based on baseline respiratory amplitude. If it is difficult to ascertain the baseline amplitude because of respiratory variability, then the apnea is terminated with a marked increase in amplitude, or if there is desaturation, with an increase of 2% in saturation level. Scoring criteria include all of the following:

- Thermal sensor drops 90% or more below baseline.
- Duration lasts 10 seconds or more (with at least 90% with reduced amplitude that marks apnea).

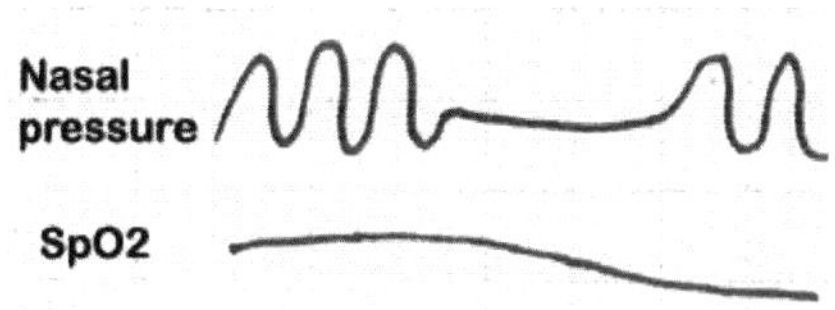

The degree of inspiratory effort determines the classification of apneas (if they also meet scoring criteria):

- Obstructive: Inspiratory effort continues or increases throughout the apneic period.
- Central: Inspiratory effort is absent during apneic period.
- Mixed: Inspiratory effort is absent for the initial apneic period but resumes during the second half of the apneic period.

SCORING HYPOPNEAS

Scoring hypopneas is similar to scoring apneas. The beginning and ending points for hypopnea are scored as apneas, from the nadir of the preceding breath to the beginning of the next normal breath, based on respiratory amplitude, or with a marked increase in respiratory amplitude or an increase of 2% in saturation (if desaturation occurs). Scoring criteria include all of the following:

- Nasal pressure (or alternative sensor): Excursions drop 30% or more from baseline.
- Duration: There are 10 seconds or more (with at least 90% with reduced amplitude that mark hypopnea).
- Oxygen saturation (SpO2): There is a 4% or more desaturation from baseline.

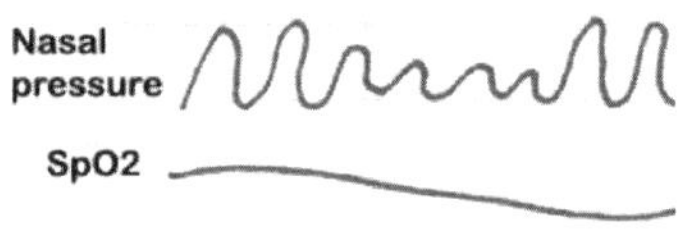

Alternative scoring criteria:

- Nasal pressure (or alternative sensor): Excursions drop 50% or more from baseline.
- Duration: There are 10 seconds or more (with at least 90% with reduced amplitude that mark hypopnea).
- SpO2: There is a 3% or more desaturation from baseline, or the event is associated with arousal.

The technologist should note which criteria are used to score hypopneas.

Scoring RERA and Hypoventilation

Respiratory effort–related arousal (RERA) occurs when the airway narrows during sleep, usually indicated by snoring. Although the constricted airway does not result in apnea or hypopnea, it does cause a brief arousal. Criteria for scoring RERA include the following: The sequence of respirations indicates increased respiratory effort or flattening of nasal pressure waveforms with a duration of 10 seconds or more, leading to an arousal from sleep (if not meeting criteria for apnea or hypopnea). Scoring is most effective if done in conjunction with esophageal pressure sensors, although nasal pressure/inductance plethysmography can also be used for scoring.

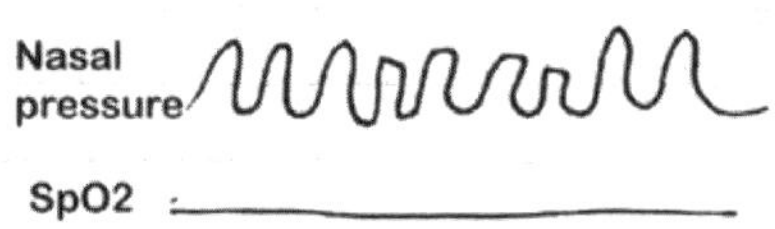

Hypoventilation is based on $PaCO_2$ scores on awakening and not on persistent desaturation. The use of other sensors is not considered adequate to determine hypoventilation. Criteria include the following: The $PaCO_2$ level (immediately after awakening) increases 10 mm Hg or more as compared to the baseline awake/supine value.

Cheyne-Stokes Respirations

Cheyne-Stokes respirations are periodic breathing characterized by periods of apnea, alternating with rapid respirations that increase in intensity and then decrease in a crescendo-to-decrescendo pattern. Pulse oximetry shows a wave-like waveform as saturation begins to fall during the apneic period and then rises after the periods of rapid respirations. Cheyne-Stokes breathing is common before death but can also occur with central nervous system damage (e.g., brain tumor, traumatic brain injury, strokes), hyperventilation, and heart failure. Criteria for scoring Cheyne-Stokes respirations include three or more consecutive cycles of a crescendo-to-decrescendo breathing pattern and one of the following:

- Cycles that persist for 10 or more consecutive minutes
- Five central apneas or central hypopneas per hour of sleep

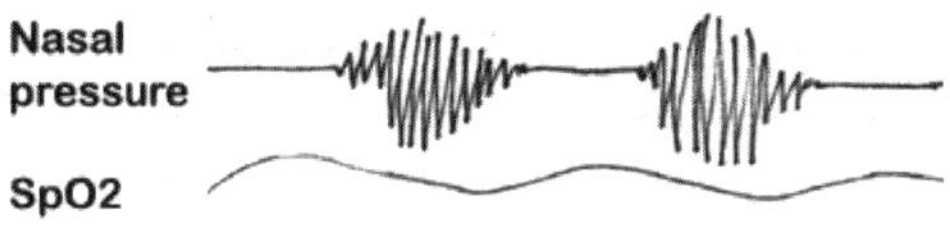

Scoring Pediatric Apneas

Scoring pediatric apneas uses the criteria listed below. This scoring for respiratory events is used for infants and children up to 18 years of age, although some centers may score adolescents 13 years of age or older, using adult criteria, depending on their size and development.

Obstructive sleep apnea (OSA)	All of the following: Duration: Two or more missed respirations (or duration of two respirations based on baseline recordings); duration is measured from end of last preceding normal breath to beginning of next normal breath. Amplitude: There is a 90% or more decrease for 90% or more of events compared to baseline. Inspiratory effort continues or increases throughout the apneic period.
Central sleep apnea	One of the following: Duration is 20 or more seconds. Duration is two or more missed respirations (or equivalent), associated with arousal, awakening, or desaturation of 3% or more.
Mixed sleep apnea	Same as scoring for OSA except inspiratory effort is absent initially but resumes before the apneic event terminates.

Scoring Pediatric Hypopneas, Periodic Breathing, and Hypoventilation

Pediatric hypopneas are scored using nasal pressure sensors, although thermal sensors may be substituted, using the same criteria, if necessary as long as the signal quality is adequate. Respiratory effort-related arousals (RERAs) must be scored with an esophageal sensor. Criteria for scoring pediatric hypopneas include all of the following:

- Nasal pressure: Amplitude decreases 50% or more as compared to baseline.
- Duration: There are two or more respirations (or equivalent duration based on baseline) with a decrease in nasal pressure, persisting for 90% or more of the event.
- Arousal, awakening, or 3% or more desaturation occurs.

Periodic breathing criteria include three or more episodes of central apnea, persisting for 3 seconds or more with 20 seconds or less of normal breathing between events.

Hypoventilation criteria include 25% of total sleep time is spent with carbon dioxide more than 50 mm Hg (according to transcutaneous PCO_2 or $etCO_2$ sensors).

Scoring Pediatric Respiratory Effort–Related Arousals

Pediatric respiratory effort–related arousals (RERAs) must be scored with adequate esophageal or nasal pressure signals. RERAs do not cause apneas or hypopneas but do restrict airways, resulting in arousal. Criteria are based on the type of sensor and must include all of the following:

Nasal pressure	There is a 50% or more decrease in amplitude from baseline.
	Nasal pressure waveforms flatten.
	There is evidence of snoring, nosing respirations, increased PCO2, or observable increased respiratory effort.
	Duration is two or more respirations (or equivalent duration of two respirations based on baseline recordings).
Esophageal pressure	Inspiratory effort increases during event.
	There is evidence of snoring, nosing respirations, increased PCO2, or observable increased respiratory effort.
	Duration is two or more respirations (or equivalent duration of two respirations based on baseline recordings).

Scoring Movements

PLMS

Periodic limb movements of sleep (PLMS) are scored as events or series:

- Event: An event ranges in duration from 0.5–10 seconds with an increased amplitude on electromyogram (EMG) of 8 microvolts or more. Timing of the event begins at the point of an 8-microvolt increase on EMG above the resting EMG and ends with a period lasting 0.5 seconds or more during which the EMG does not increase more than 2 microvolts above the resting EMG.
- Series: A series requires four or more leg consecutive movements with the time between movements, ranging from a minimum of 5 seconds to a maximum of 90 seconds. Leg movements involving both legs are counted as one movement if they occur within 5 seconds of each other.

Leg movements are not scored if they occur 0.5 seconds before or 0.5 seconds after an episode of apnea or hypopnea. Leg movements and arousals are considered as associated events if one occurs within 0.5 seconds after the end of the other, regardless of which one occurred first.

ALMA and HFTs

Alternating leg muscle activation (ALMA) occurs with rapid alternating activation of electromyograms (EMGs) in the lower extremities. ALMA may be associated with periodic leg movements of sleep. An ALMA series requires at least four ALMAs at a minimum frequency of 0.5 Hz and a maximum frequency of 3.0 Hz. Duration usually ranges from 100–500 milliseconds. ALMAs are considered benign, do not require treatment, and are unrelated to sleep disorders.

Hypnagogic foot tremors (HFTs) are tremors that occur during sleep onset. HFTs may occur in one or both feet. HFTs are most common in stage W but may continue into stages 1 and 2 non-REM sleep. HFTs are scored with a minimum of four EMG bursts in the frequency range of 0.3–4.0 Hz. Duration ranges from 250–1000 milliseconds.

EFM

Scoring excessive fragmentary myoclonus (EFM), which is twitching movements of the fingers, toes, and mouth that may occur during stage W as well as non-REM and REM sleep, requires that the activity continues for at least 20 minutes of non-REM sleep with at least five electromyographic (EMG) potentials per minute. This twitching is similar to that found in REM sleep, but it is more regular. The duration of a burst of activity usually is 150 milliseconds or less, although it may exceed 150 milliseconds if twitching is obvious. Jerking motions are not associated with EFM. In many cases, the twitching is not observable, but activity may be noted on the EMG and the chin EMG. EFM appears to be benign.

Bruxism

Scoring bruxism, which is grinding of the teeth, is done with masseter electrodes as well as with a chin electromyogram (cEMG). Bruxism may occur with sustained clenching, tonic contractions, or with rhythmic muscle activity, which comprises a series of brief contractions. Some clenching of the teeth is normal during sleep, but excessive grinding of the teeth or jaw clenching may cause damage to the teeth and disrupt sleep. Requirements for coding bruxism include the following:

- Phasic (brief) or tonic (sustained) increases in cEMG activity at least two times the amplitude of a background cEMG.
    - Phasic: Sequence of at least three with duration of each 0.25–2 seconds
    - Tonic: Duration of 2 seconds or more
- A new bruxism event is scored only after 3 or more seconds of a stable background cEMG.
- Audible scoring: Two or more tooth grinding events a night (in the absence of epilepsy)

RBD

Scoring a REM sleep behavior disorder (RBD) requires a polysomnogram (PSG) and a video, audio, or clinical history of REM occurring without atonia or with excessive muscle activity. Some transient muscle activity, usually involving the muscles of the hands, feet, or mouth, often occurs during REM sleep. Some large muscle activity may also occur but does not involve muscle activity across joints. With RBD, a baseline chin electromyogram (cEMG) and an anterior tibialis EMG (atEMG) may have a slightly higher frequency than usually occurs because the state of atonia that normally occurs is missing. Scoring RBD during REM sleep uses the following criteria:

- Sustained muscle activity: REM epoch with 50% or more increased cEMG activity
- Excessive transient muscle activity: 50% or more of ten mini-epochs (3-second intervals in a 30-second epoch); includes bursts of muscle activity, usually 0.1–5.0 seconds in duration with amplitude increased fourfold over baseline EMG activity

RMD

Scoring rhythmic movement disorder (RMD), which is very common in infants, beginning at about 6 months of age and continuing until 2–3 years of age, is dependent on the criteria listed below. The incidence after age 5 is rare unless a patient has an injury to the central nervous system. RMD often includes rocking, head banging, or head rolling, although some children may have leg banging and body rolling as well. RMD most often occurs during stage W when the patient is very drowsy or during stage 1 non-REM sleep. These rhythmic movements may be accompanied by humming. Criteria for scoring RMD include the following:

- There are clusters of four or more rhythmic movements.
- Amplitude of each burst is double background EMG activity.
- The frequency ranges between a minimum of 0.5 Hz to a maximum of 2.0 Hz.

A video synchronized with the polysomnogram is required for diagnosis.

Scoring Cardiac Events

Normal Conduction of the Heart

The normal conduction of the heart has four stages:

- Generation of impulse at the sinoatrial (SA) node (primary pacemaker) located at the junction of the right atrium and superior vena cava: The electrical impulse travels in the cells of the atria along internodal pathways, causing electrical stimulation and contraction of the atria.
- Atrioventricular (AV) node conduction of impulse: This occurs when the impulses from the SA node reach the AV node in the right atrial wall near the tricuspid valve. There is a slight delay (about one-tenth of a second), allowing the atria to empty.
- AV bundle (bundle of His) conduction: The AV node relays the impulse to the ventricles through the AV bundle, which are specialized conduction cells in the ventricular septum that branch to the right and left ventricles, carrying the electrical impulse.
- Purkinje fiber conduction: The impulses are conducted down the AV bundles to the base of the heart where they divide into Purkinje fibers, which stimulate the myocardial cells to contract the ventricles.

Scoring Cardiac Events

Scoring cardiac events is done with the electrocardiogram (ECG). When evaluating the ECG to determine if arrhythmias are present, the following steps ensure a systematic review, viewing 6–10-second recordings:

- Note the absence or presence of P waves: Absence usually means an arrhythmia is not atrial (except with atrial fibrillation or atrial flutter).
- Note the absence, presence, or change in the QRS sequence: Absence indicates AV block or ventricular abnormalities (fibrillation or asystole).
- Note the relationship between the P wave and the QRS complex:
    - P:QRS ratio of 1:1 with more P waves than QRS complexes indicates AV block.
    - P:QRS ratio of less than 1:1 with more QRS complexes than P waves indicates junctional or ventricular arrhythmia.
- Note the P-R and QRS intervals:
    - A shortened P-R interval indicates junctional beat or accessory pathway syndrome.
    - An increased P-R interval indicates AV block.
    - A widened QRS complex indicates bundle branch block (BBB), a beat originating in the ventricles, or aberrant supraventricular beat.
- Note the regularity of rhythm by examining P-P and R-R intervals.
- Note the heart rate.

HEART RATE AND RHYTHM

Determining the heart rate can be done in a number of ways but estimating with a short recording (< 30 seconds) should only be done if cardiac rhythm is essentially regular. The sleep technologist should compare 30-second recordings with 6–10-second recordings to determine if there are abnormalities. The normal heart rate varies considerably, ranging from 60–100 beats/min. Methods of counting include the following:

- Count beats for 30-second intervals and multiply x 2.
- Count beats for 14-second intervals and multiply x 4.
- Count the number of R-R intervals in a 6-second reading and multiply by 10.

Heart rhythm should be regular. A normal sinus rhythm is characterized by a P wave and QRS complex present with each beat and having the same appearance:

- P:QRS ratio: 1:1
- P-R interval: 0.12–0.20 seconds
- QRS interval: 0.04–0.11 seconds

SINUS BRADYCARDIA

Sinus bradycardia is caused by a decreased rate of impulses from the sinus node. The pulse and electrocardiogram (ECG) usually appear normal except for a slower rate.

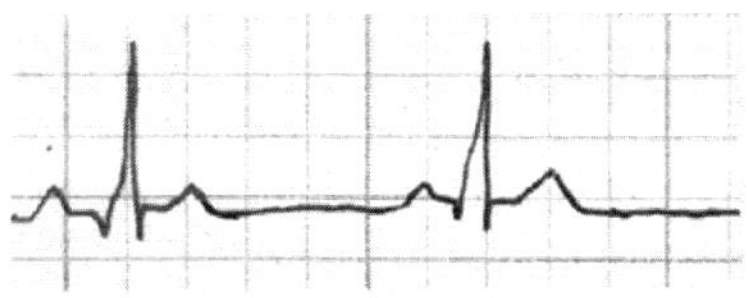

Sinus bradycardia is characterized by a regular pulse of less than 50–60 beats/min with P waves in front of QRS complexes, which are usually normal in shape and duration. The P-R interval is 0.12–0.20 seconds; the QRS interval is 0.04–0.11 seconds; and the P:QRS ratio is 1:1. Sinus bradycardia may be caused by a number of factors:

- Hypotension and a decrease in oxygenation
- Conditions that lower the body's metabolic needs, such as hypothermia or sleep
- Medications, such as calcium channel blockers and β-blockers
- Vagal stimulation that may result from vomiting, suctioning, or defecating
- Increased intracranial pressure
- Myocardial infarction

Sinus bradycardia is scored during sleep with a sustained heart rate of less than 40 beats/min for patients 6 years of age or more through adulthood.

SINUS TACHYCARDIA

Sinus tachycardia occurs when the sinus node impulse increases in frequency. Sinus tachycardia is characterized by a regular pulse of 100 beats/min or more with P waves before QRS complexes but sometimes a part of a preceding T wave. QRS is usually of normal shape and duration (0.04–0.11 seconds) but may have consistent irregularity. The P-R interval is 0.12–0.20 seconds, and P:QRS ratio is 1:1. The rapid pulse decreases diastolic filling time and causes reduced cardiac output with resultant hypotension. Acute pulmonary edema may result from the decreased ventricular filling if untreated. Sinus tachycardia may be caused by a number of factors:

- Acute blood loss, shock, hypovolemia, and anemia
- Sinus arrhythmia and hypovolemic heart failure
- Hypermetabolic conditions, fever, and infection
- Exertion/exercise and anxiety
- Medications, such as sympathomimetic drugs

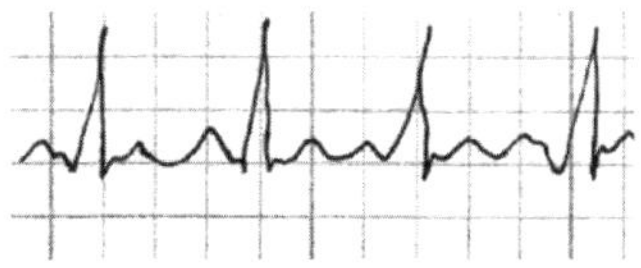

Sinus tachycardia is scored during sleep if there is a sustained heart rate of 90 beat/min or more in adults.

SUPRAVENTRICULAR TACHYCARDIA

Supraventricular tachycardia (> 100 beats/min) may have a sudden onset and result in congestive heart failure. Rates may increase to 200–300 beats/min. Supraventricular tachycardia originates in the atria rather than the ventricles but is controlled by the tissue in the area of the atrioventricular node rather than the sinoatrial node. Rhythm is usually rapid but regular. The P wave is present but may not be clearly defined as it may be obscured by the preceding T wave, and the QRS complex appears normal. The P-R interval is 0.12–0.20 seconds, and the QRS interval is 0.04–0.11 seconds with a P:QRS ratio of 1:1. Supraventricular tachycardia may be episodic with periods of normal heart rate and rhythm between episodes, so it is often referred to as paroxysmal supraventricular tachycardia.

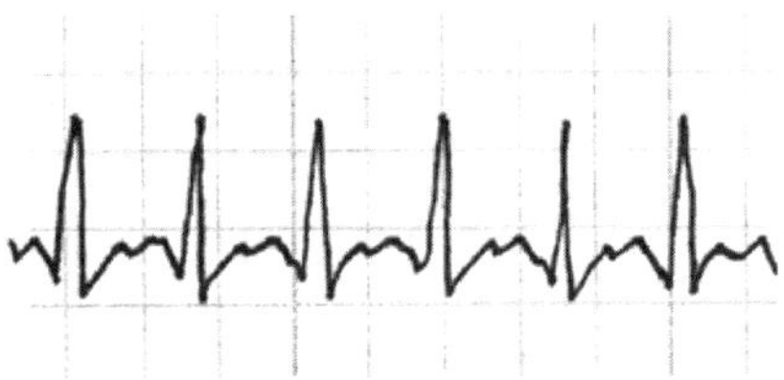

PREMATURE ATRIAL CONTRACTIONS

Premature atrial contractions are essentially extra beats precipitated by an electrical impulse to the atrium before the sinus node impulse. The extra beat may be caused by alcohol, caffeine, nicotine, hypervolemia, hypokalemia, hypermetabolic conditions, atrial ischemia or infarction. Characteristics include an irregular pulse because of extra P waves; the shape and duration of the QRS complex is usually normal (0.04–0.11 seconds) but may be abnormal; the P-R interval remains between 0.12–0.20; and the P:QRS ratio is 1:1. Rhythm is irregular with varying P-P and R-R intervals. Premature atrial contractions can occur in an essentially healthy heart and are not usually cause for concern unless they are frequent (> 6/hr) and cause severe palpitations. In that case, atrial fibrillation should be suspected.

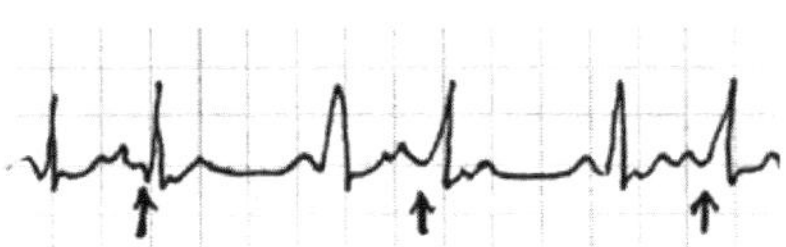

Sinus Arrhythmia

Sinus arrhythmia results from irregular impulses from the sinus node, often paradoxical (increasing with inspiration and decreasing with expiration) because of stimulation of the vagus nerve during inspiration and rarely causes a negative hemodynamic effect. These cyclic changes in the pulse during respiration are quite common in both children and young adults and often lessen with age but may persist in some adults. Sinus arrhythmia can, in some cases, relate to heart or valvular disease and may be increased with vagal stimulation for suctioning, vomiting, or defecating. Sinus arrhythmia is characterized by: a regular pulse of 50–100 beats/min; P waves in front of QRS complexes with a duration of 0.4–0.11 seconds; a shape of the QRS complex that is usually normal; a P-R interval of 0.12–0.20 seconds; and a P:QRS ratio of 1:1.

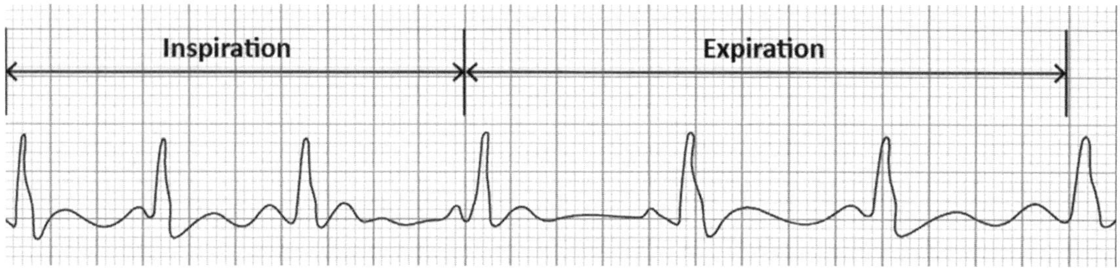

Atrial Flutter

Atrial flutter occurs when the atrial rate is faster, usually 250–400 beats/min, than the atrioventricular (AV) node conduction rate; thus, not all of the beats are conducted into the ventricles, which are effectively blocked at the AV node, preventing ventricular fibrillation, although some extra ventricular impulses may go though. Atrial flutter is caused by the same conditions that cause atrial fibrillation: coronary artery disease, valvular disease, pulmonary disease, heavy alcohol ingestion, and cardiac surgery. Atrial fibrillation is characterized by atrial rates of 250–400 beats/min with ventricular rates of 75–150 beats/min; ventricular rates are usually regular. P waves are saw-toothed (referred to as F waves); the QRS complex shape and duration of 0.4–0.11 seconds are usually normal; the P-R interval may be hard to calculate because of F waves; and the P:QRS ratio is 2–4:1. Symptoms include chest pain, dyspnea, and hypotension.

Atrial Fibrillation

Atrial fibrillation is rapid, disorganized atrial beats that are ineffective in emptying the atria, so that blood pools and can lead to thrombus formation and emboli. The ventricular rate increases with a decreased stroke volume, and cardiac output decreases with increased myocardial ischemia, resulting in palpitations and fatigue. Atrial fibrillation is caused by coronary artery disease, valvular disease, pulmonary disease, heavy alcohol ingestion, and cardiac surgery. Atrial fibrillation is characterized by a very irregular pulse with an atrial rate of 300–600 beats/min and a ventricular rate of 120–200 beats/min; the shape and duration (0.4–0.11 seconds) of the QRS complex is usually normal. Fibrillatory (F) waves are seen instead of P waves. The P-R interval cannot be measured, and the P:QRS ratio is highly variable. This is scored as atrial fibrillation during sleep with irregularly irregular ventricular rhythm and varying rapid oscillations replacing P waves.

Sinus Pause

Sinus pause occurs when the sinus node fails to function properly to stimulate heart contractions and the P wave, so there is a pause on the electrocardiogram recording that may persist for a few seconds to minutes, depending on the severity of the dysfunction. A prolonged pause may be difficult to differentiate from cardiac arrest, so the technologist should alert medical personnel if the pause persists more than a few seconds. During the sinus pause, the P wave, QRS complex, and the P-R and QRS intervals are all absent. The P:QRS ratio is 1:1, and the rhythm is irregular. The pulse rate may vary widely, usually 60–100 beat/min. Patients frequently complain of dizziness or syncope. Score asystole for pauses of more than 3 seconds for ages 6 through adulthood.

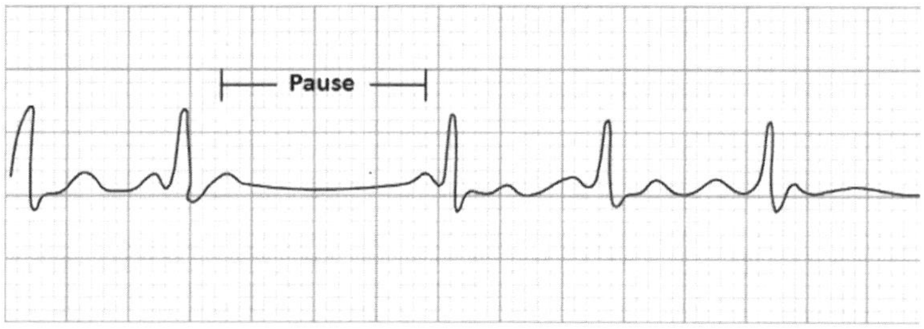

Premature Junctional Contractions

Premature junctional contractions occur when a premature impulse starts at the atrioventricular (AV) node before the next normal sinus impulse reaches the AV node. The area around the AV node is the junction, and dysrhythmias that arise from that are called junctional dysrhythmias. Premature junctional contractions are similar to premature atrial contractions and generally require no treatment, although they may be an indication of digoxin toxicity. The electrocardiogram may appear basically normal with an early QRS complex that is normal in shape and duration (0.4–0.11 seconds). The P wave may be absent, precede, be part of, or follow the QRS complex with a P-R interval of 0.12 seconds. The P:QRS ratio may vary from less than 1:1 to 1:1 (with an inverted P wave). Rhythm is usually regular at a heart rate of 40–60 beats/min. Significant symptoms related to premature junctional contractions are rare.

Junctional Rhythms

Junctional rhythms occur when the atrioventricular (AV) node becomes the pacemaker of the heart because the sinus node is depressed from increased vagal tone, or a block at the AV node prevents sinus node impulses from being transmitted. While the sinus node normally sends impulses of 60–100 beats/min, the AV node junction usually sends impulses at 40–60 beats/min. The QRS complex is of usual shape and duration (0.4–0.11 seconds). The P wave may be inverted and may be absent, hidden, or come after the QRS complex. If the P wave precedes the QRS complex, the P-R interval is less than 0.12 seconds. The P:QRS ratio is less than 1:1 or 1:1. The junctional escape rhythm is a protective mechanism preventing asystole with failure of the sinus node. An accelerated junctional rhythm is similar, but the heart rate is 60–100 beats/min. Junctional tachycardia occurs with a heart rate of over 100 beats/min.

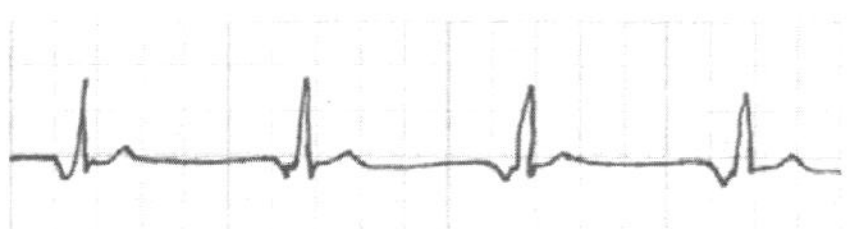

PVCs

Premature ventricular contractions (PVCs) are those in which the impulse begins in the ventricles and conducts through them before the next sinus impulse. The ectopic QRS complexes may vary in shape, depending on whether there is one site (unifocal), or more (multifocal), that is stimulating the ectopic beats. PVCs usually cause no morbidity unless there is underlying cardiac disease or an acute myocardial infarction. PVCs are characterized by an irregular heart beat; a QRS complex that is 0.12 seconds or more and oddly shaped; a P wave that may be absent or may precede or follow the QRS complex; a P-R interval of less than 0.12 seconds if the P wave is present; and a P:QRS ratio of 0–1:1. Short-term therapy may include lidocaine, but PVCs are often not treated in otherwise healthy people. PVCs may be precipitated by caffeine, nicotine, or alcohol. Because PVCs may occur with any supraventricular dysrhythmia, the underlying rhythm (e.g., atrial fibrillation) must be noted as well as the PVCs.

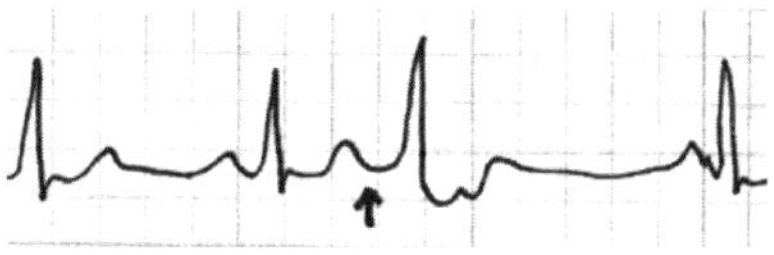

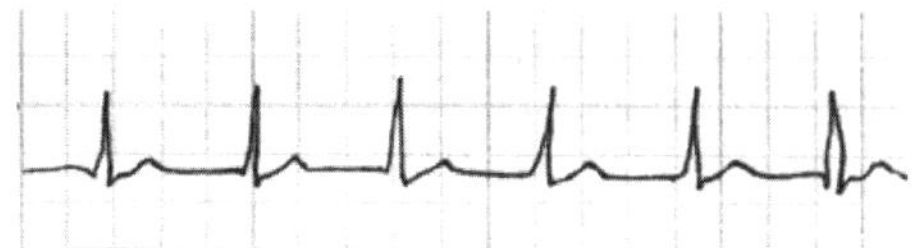

Ventricular Tachycardia

Ventricular tachycardia is three or more premature ventricular contractions (PVCs) in a row with a ventricular rate of 100–200 beats/min. Ventricular tachycardia may be triggered by the same things as PVCs and is often related to underlying coronary artery disease, but the rapid rate of contractions make ventricular tachycardia dangerous as the ineffective beats may render the person unconscious with no palpable pulse. A detectable rate is usually regular, and the QRS complex is 0.12 seconds or more and abnormally shaped. The P wave may be undetectable with an irregular P-R interval if the P wave is present. The P:QRS ratio is often difficult to ascertain because of the absence of P waves.

Narrow-Complex and Wide-Complex Tachycardias

For scoring purposes, tachycardias are scored as narrow complex or wide complex. Wide and narrow refer to the configuration of the QRS complex:

- Wide-complex tachycardia: About 80% of cases of wide-complex tachycardias are caused by ventricular tachycardia. Wide-complex tachycardia originates at some point below the atrioventricular node and may be associated with palpitations, dyspnea, anxiety, and cardiac arrest. Patients may exhibit diaphoresis. It is scored as a wide-complex tachycardia with three or more consecutive beats at a heart rate of 100 beat/min or more and a QRS complex duration of 0.12 seconds or more.
- Narrow-complex tachycardia: Narrow-complex tachycardias are associated with palpitations, dyspnea, and peripheral edema. Narrow-complex tachycardias are generally supraventricular in origin. They are scored as a narrow-complex tachycardia with three or more consecutive beats at a heart rate of 100 beats/min or more and a QRS complex duration of less than 0.12 seconds.

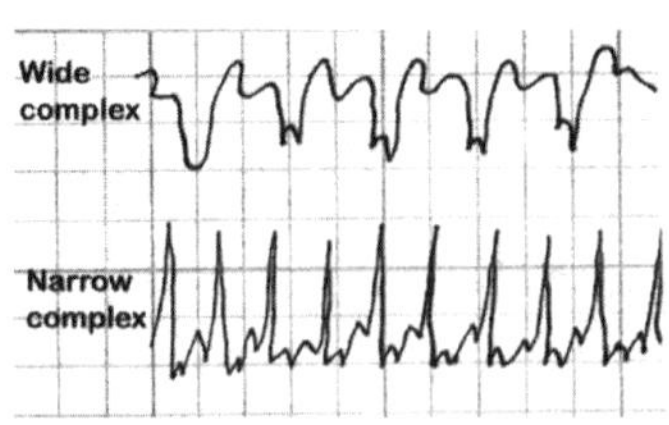

Ventricular Fibrillation

Ventricular fibrillation is a rapid, very irregular ventricular rate of more than 300 beats/min with no atrial activity observable on the electrocardiogram (ECG), caused by disorganized electrical activity in the ventricles. The QRS complex is not recognizable as the ECG shows irregular undulations. The causes are the same as for ventricular tachycardia (e.g., alcohol, caffeine, nicotine, underlying coronary disease), and it may result if ventricular tachycardia is not treated. It may also result from an electrical shock or congenital disorder, such as Brugada syndrome. Ventricular fibrillation is accompanied by a lack of a palpable pulse, audible pulse, and respirations and is immediately life-threatening without defibrillation. After emergency defibrillation, the cause should be identified and limited. Mortality is high if ventricular fibrillation occurs as part of a myocardial infarction.

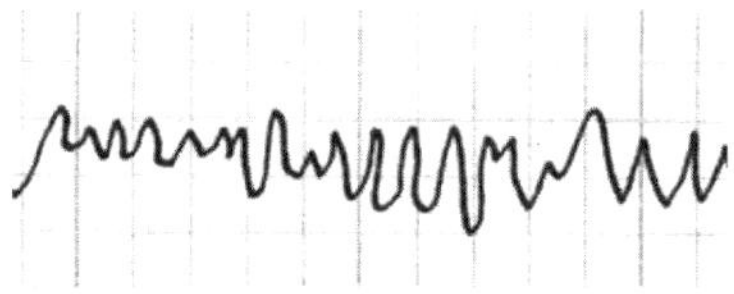

Idioventricular Rhythm

Idioventricular rhythm (or ventricular escape rhythm) occurs when the Purkinje fibers below the atrioventricular (AV) node create an impulse. This may occur if the sinus node fails to fire or if there is blockage at the AV node so that the impulse does not go through. Idioventricular rhythm is characterized by a regular ventricular rate of 20–40 beats/min. Rates over 40 beats/min are called accelerated idioventricular rhythm. The P wave is missing, and the QRS complex has a very bizarre and abnormal shape with a duration of 0.12 seconds or more. The low ventricular rate may cause a decrease in cardiac output, often making the patient lose consciousness. In other patients, the idioventricular rhythm may not be associated with reduced cardiac output.

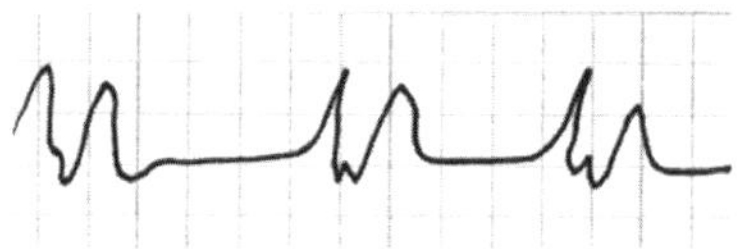

Ventricular Asystole

Ventricular asystole is the absence of an audible heartbeat, palpable pulse, and respirations, a condition often referred to as "flat-lining" or "cardiac arrest." While the electrocardiogram may show some P waves initially, the QRS complex is absent although there may be an occasional QRS "escape beat." Cardiopulmonary resuscitation is required with intubation for ventilation and establishment of an intravenous line for fluids. Without immediate treatment, the patient will suffer from severe hypoxia and brain death within minutes. Identifying the cause is critical for the patient's survival and could include hypoxia, acidosis, electrolyte imbalance, hypothermia, or drug overdose. Even with immediate treatment, the prognosis is poor, and ventricular asystole is often a sign of impending death.

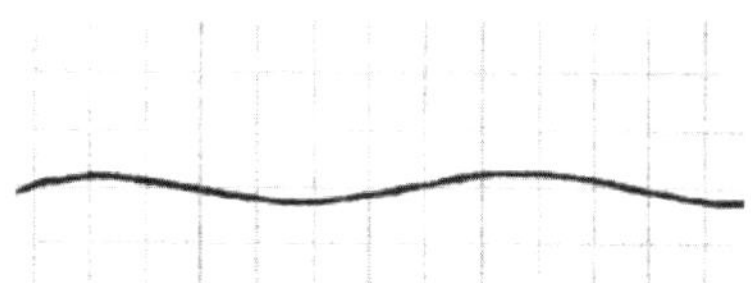

First-Degree Atrioventricular Block

First-degree atrioventricular (AV) block occurs when the atrial impulses are conducted through the AV node to the ventricles at a rate that is slower than normal. While the P wave and the QRS complex are usually normal, the P-R interval is 0.20 seconds or more, and the P:QRS ratio is 1:1. A narrow QRS complex indicates a conduction abnormality only in the AV node, but a widened QRS complex indicates associated damage to the bundle branches as well. Chronic first-degree AV block may be caused by fibrosis or sclerosis of the conduction system related to coronary artery disease, valvular disease, and cardiac myopathies and carries little morbidity. Acute first-degree AV block, on the other hand, is of much more concern and may be related to digoxin toxicity, β-blockers, amiodarone, myocardial infarction, hyperkalemia, or edema related to valvular surgery.

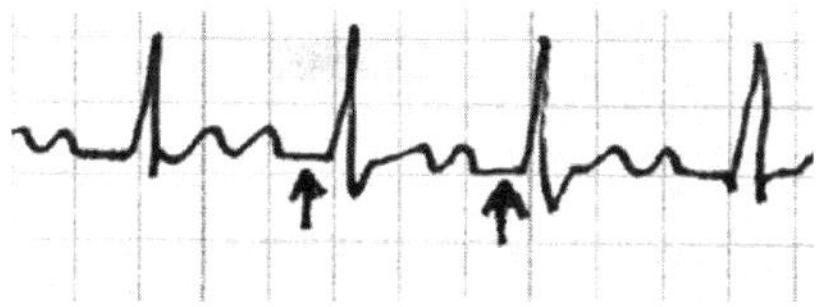

Second-Degree Atrioventricular Block, Type I

Second-degree atrioventricular (AV) block occurs when some of the atrial beats are blocked. Second-degree AV block is further subdivided, according to patterns of block. With a Mobitz type I block (Wenckebach), each atrial impulse in a group of beats is conducted at a lengthened interval until one fails to conduct (the P-R interval progressively increases), so there are more P waves than QRS complexes, but the QRS complex is usually of normal shape and duration. The sinus node functions at a regular rate, so the P-P interval is regular, but the R-R interval usually shortens with each impulse. The P:QRS ratio varies, such as 3:2, 4:3, and 5:4. This type of block by itself usually does not cause significant morbidity unless associated with inferior wall myocardial infarction.

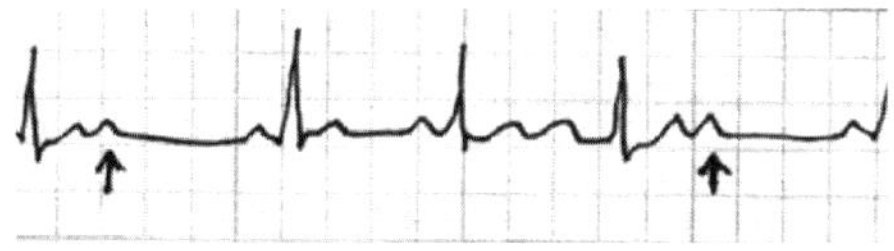

Second-Degree Atrioventricular Block, Type II and 2:1 Block

Second-degree atrioventricular (AV) block, type II (Mobitz), is characterized by only some of the atrial impulses conducted unpredictably through the AV node to the ventricles, and the block always occurs below the AV node in the bundle of His, the bundle branches, or the Purkinje fibers. The P-R intervals are the same if impulses are conducted, and the QRS complex is usually widened. The P:QRS ratio varies from 2:1, 3:1, and 4:1. Type II block is more dangerous than type I because it may progress to complete AV block and may produce Stokes-Adams syncope. Additionally, if the block is at the Purkinje fibers, there is no escape impulse. Usually, a transcutaneous cardiac pacemaker and defibrillator should be at the bedside. Symptoms may include chest pain if the heart block is precipitated by myocarditis or myocardial ischemia. With a 2:1 block every other atrial impulse (P:QRS ratio of 2:1) is conducted through the AV node.

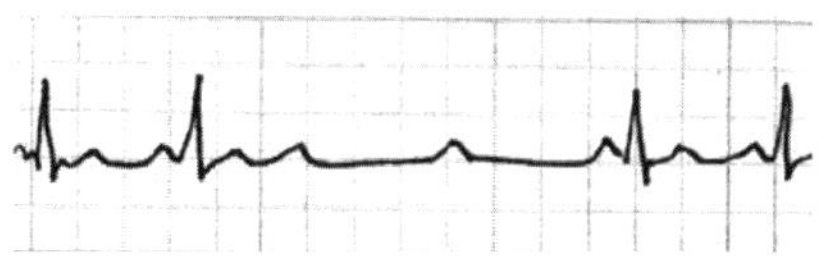

Third-Degree Atrioventricular Block

Third-degree atrioventricular (AV) block is characterized by more P waves than QRS complexes with no clear relationship between them and an atrial rate two to three times the pulse rate, so the P-R interval is irregular. If the sinoatrial node malfunctions, the AV node fires at a lower rate, and if the AV node malfunctions, the pacemaker site in the ventricles takes over at a bradycardic rate; thus, with complete AV block, the heart still contracts, but often ineffectually. With this type of block, the atrial P (sinus rhythm or atrial fibrillation) and the ventricular QRS (ventricular escape rhythm) are stimulated by different impulses, so there is AV dissociation. The heart may compensate at rest but cannot keep pace with exertion. The resultant bradycardia may cause congestive heart failure, fainting, or even sudden death, and usually conduction abnormalities slowly worsen. Symptoms include dyspnea, chest pain, and hypotension, which are treated with intravenous atropine. Transcutaneous pacing may be needed. Complete persistent AV block normally requires implanted pacemakers, usually dual chamber.

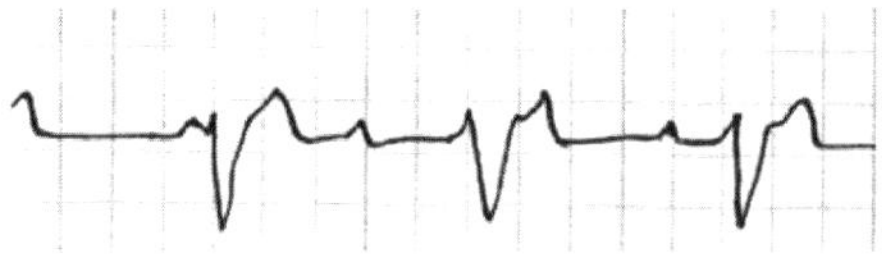

Right Bundle Branch Block and Left Bundle Branch Block

A right bundle branch block (RBBB) occurs when conduction is blocked in the right bundle branch that carries impulses from the Bundle of His to the right ventricle. The impulse travels through the left ventricle instead, and then reaches the right ventricle, but this causes a slight delay in contraction of the right ventricle. A RBBB is characterized by normal P waves (as the right atrium still contract appropriately), but the QRS complex is widened and notched (rabbit-eared) in lead V1, which is a reflection of the asynchronous ventricular contraction. The PR interval is normal or prolonged, and the QRS interval is > 0.12 seconds. P: QRS ratio remains 1:1 with regular rhythms.

A left bundle branch block (LBBB) occurs when there is a delay in conduction between the left atrium and left ventricle. It is also characterized by normal P waves, but the QRS complex may be widened with a deep S wave and interval of >0.12 seconds (in lead V1). The PR interval may be normal or prolonged. The P:QRS ratio is 1:1 and rhythm is regular.

In Lead V1:

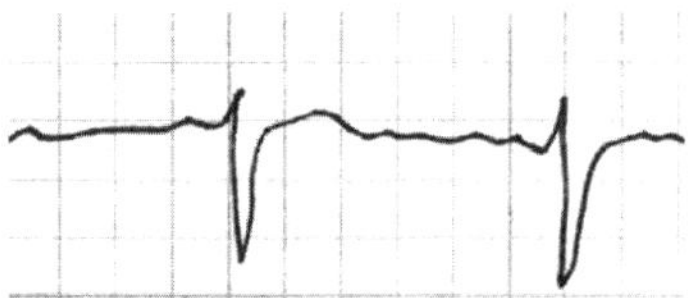

Left Bundle Branch Block

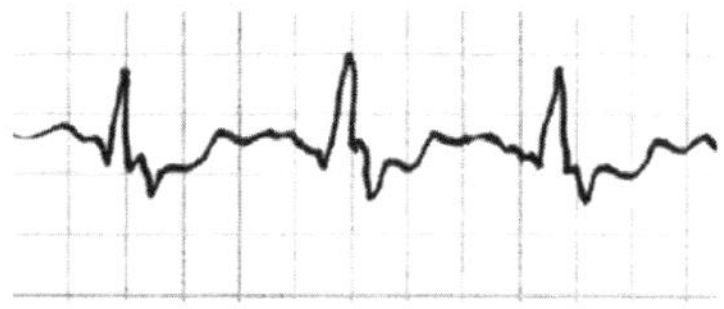

Right Bundle Branch Block

Waveform Variations

Alpha Waves

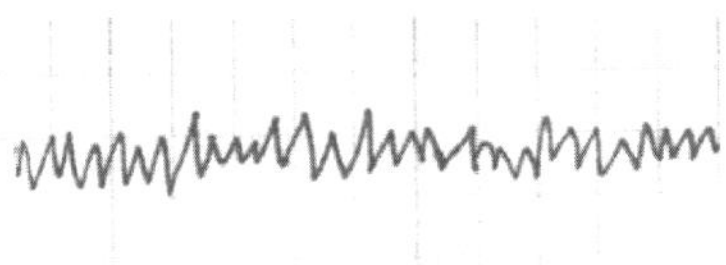

Alpha waves are 8–13 Hz frequency with an amplitude of less than 50 microvolts for adults, but often slightly slower for children and older adults. Alpha waves are slow and synchronous and are most typical at the onset of sleep when the patient is very drowsy and the eyes are closed. They also occur with deep relaxation and meditation. Alpha waves are suppressed when the eyes open. Alpha waves may also occur during arousals. Alpha waves are more noticeable in the occipital leads as they originate in the occipital cortex. Alpha-delta waves are slow alpha waves, occurring during periods of stage 3 non-REM sleep usually characterized by delta waves.

Beta Waves and Delta Waves

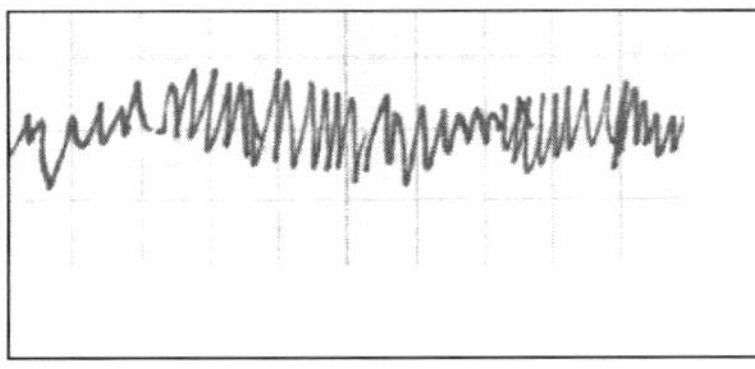	**Beta waves** are 13–35 Hz with an amplitude of less than 30 microvolts. Beta waves are present during normal wakefulness when the patient is alert.

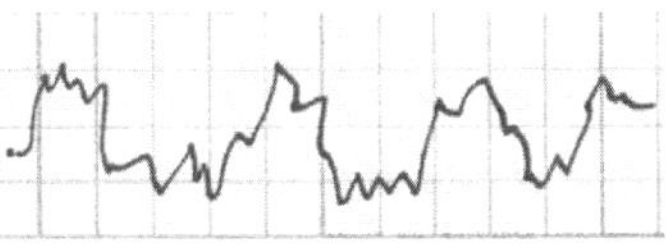	**Delta waves** are slow 1–4 Hz with a high amplitude of more than 75 microvolts and are present in stage 3 non REM (slow-wave) sleep in adults. Delta waves occur in the waking state of newborns and young children and may occur in adults who are intoxicated or have dementia or schizophrenia. Delta waves are involved in the release of human growth hormone, and patients are most deeply asleep during delta-wave activity.

Theta Waves, Sawtooth Waves, and Vertex Waves

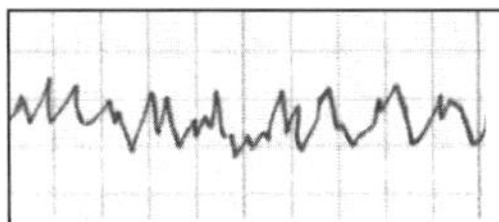	**Theta waves** are 4–6 Hz with oscillations of varying amplitude and are most easily observed with central and temporal leads. Theta waves are common during daydreaming and self-hypnotic states, occur in stage 1 non-REM sleep, and may occur during arousals.
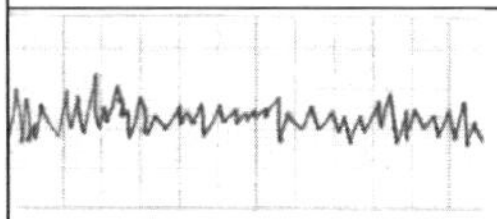	**Sawtooth waves** are notched waves in the theta range that occur during REM sleep and are most easily observed with frontal and vertex leads.
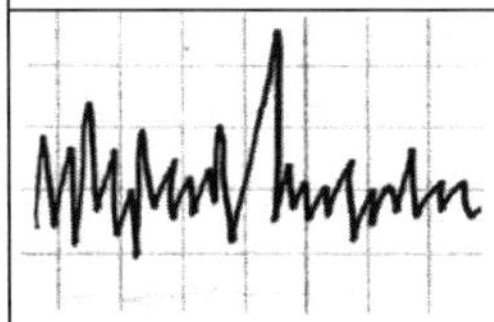	**Vertex waves** (vertex sharp transients, vertex sharp deflections, V waves) are commonly found negative deflections with amplitude usually ranging from 50–150 microvolts; they are most noticeable from vertex and frontal leads. They may have sharp contours and occur in repetitive episodes (especially in children).

Sleep Spindles and K Complexes

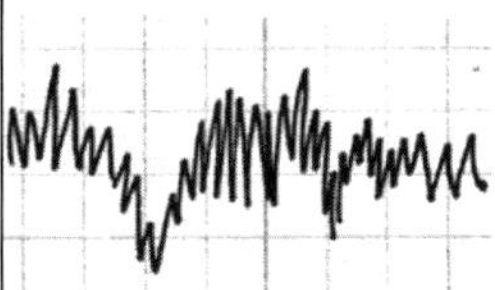	**Sleep spindles** are 12–14 Hz with an amplitude of less than 30 microvolts and a duration of 0.5–1.5 seconds, representing sudden bursts of electrical activity, usually most noticeable from central leads. They are slightly slower than alpha waves. Sleep spindles occur in sleep stages 2 and 3 non-REM but do not occur in stage 1 non-REM or in REM sleep. Sleep spindles usually indicate the onset of stage 2 non-REM sleep. Similar appearing spindles may occur with benzodiazepine use, but they can be differentiated by a higher frequency (15 Hz).
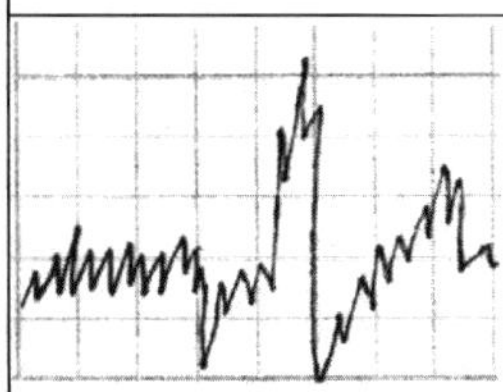	**K complexes** are sharp negative waves (usually > 100 microvolts), preceding slower positive waves, and finally smaller negative waves, persisting for more than 0.5 seconds, sometimes followed by sleep spindles. K complexes occur during stage 2 non-REM sleep, usually every 1–1.7 minutes.

Wicket Spike Waves and Benign Epileptiform Transients of Sleep or Small Sharp Spikes

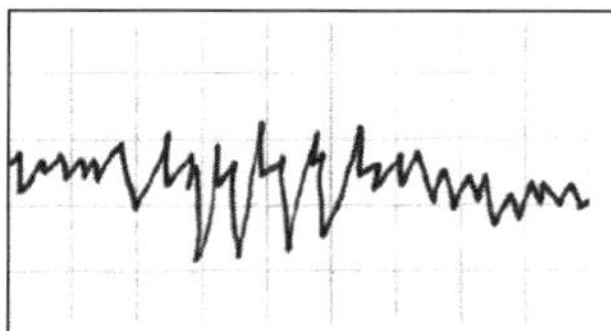	**Wicket spike waves** are 6–11 Hz frequency and occur primarily in older adults in a drowsy wake stage or stage 1 non-REM sleep. They are a normal variant and do not indicate pathology. Wicket spikes have a symmetric up and down arc and do not cross below the baseline as interictal epileptiform activity does, and they have little impact on the background electroencephalogram (EEG) reading. They may occur as single spikes or runs of spikes and are not followed by a slow wave.
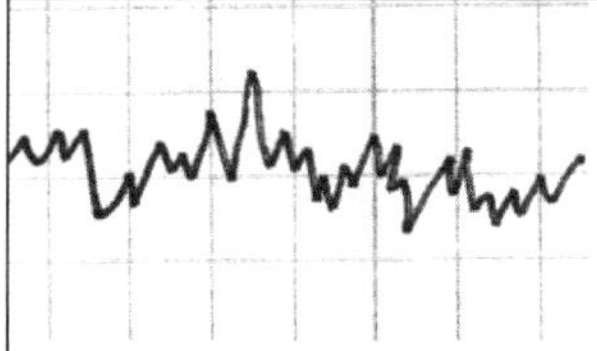	**Benign epileptiform transients of sleep** occur occasionally in stage 1 non-REM and stage 2 non-REM sleep. They are also called **small sharp spikes** because they are brief (< 50 milliseconds) with small amplitude (< 50 milliampere) and do not disrupt the background EEG.

IEA

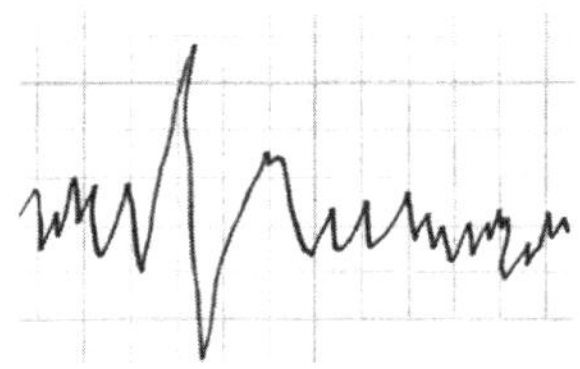

Interictal epileptiform activity (IEA) is electrical discharges that occur between epileptic seizures. IEA usually occurs in brief bursts of electrical activity rather than the prolonged activity that is more representative of actual seizures. Typically, the spikes are asymmetric, with the downward arc, crossing below the baseline and more sloping than the upward arc. There are four types, which are described below.

Sharp wave	Pointed waves that are distinct from the background electroencephalogram, lasting 70–200 milliseconds
Spike	Similar to sharp-wave discharges but duration is shorter, 20–70 milliseconds.
Spike and slow-wave complex	Spike discharge followed by a slow wave of higher amplitude
Multiple spike and slow-wave complex	Multiple spike and slow-wave complex: multiple spikes (> 2) followed by one or more slow waves

Epileptic Seizure Activity

Epileptic seizure activity is evident on the polysomnogram (PSG), often across all channels, but the presentation depends on the type of seizure. Some seizure activity, such as frontal lobe epilepsy, occurs primarily during sleep. Seizure activity is most common during non-REM sleep stages, especially stage 2 non-REM. A PSG may help to differentiate between obstructive sleep apnea syndrome (OSAS) and frontal lobe epilepsy, which can result in similar symptoms of choking and excessive daytime drowsiness. In some cases, both epilepsy and OSAS may be present. Sleep disorders may exacerbate epileptic activity. Four-channel electroencephalogram recordings are more likely to demonstrate frontal lobe epilepsy accurately than temporal lobe, which is better identified with 18 channels, so some epileptic activity may be difficult to identify. Video monitoring during PSG can help to identify seizure activity, which usually involves some degree of arousal.

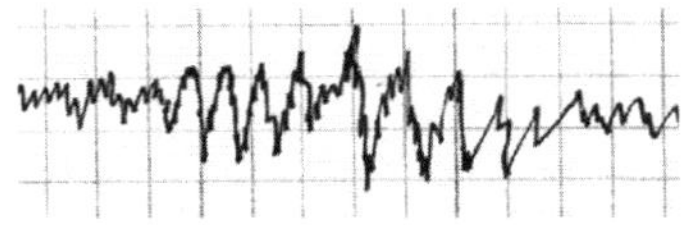

Low-Level 50–60 Hz and Electrode Popping/Chin Electromyogram

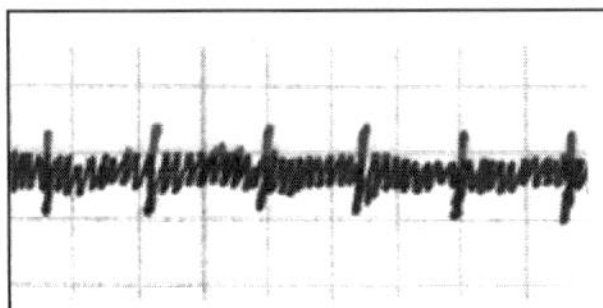	**Low-level 50–60 Hz artifacts** from power line interference, other electrical equipment, or an electrode connection are commonly found in polysomnography and are often detected in electromyogram (EMG) channels, such as the chin EMG (cEMG). Additionally, especially if related to dislodged electrodes, the electrocardiogram (ECG) signals may be evident in the cEMG channel. In the case of 60 Hz artifacts, the appearance of the cEMG recording will be very uniform.
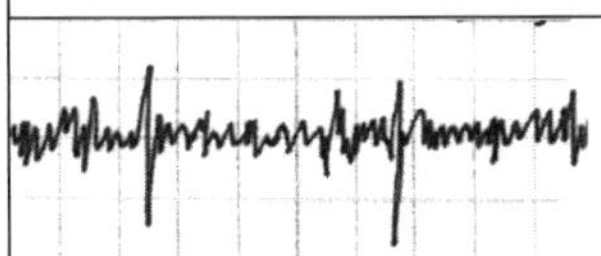	**Electrode popping** causes a series of spike-like waves that mirror respirations, usually because the electrode is loose, dirty, faulty, or pressing against bedding. ECG signals may also be evident in the cEMG recording. A tight electrode seal to the skin may prevent electrode popping.

Airflow and Respiratory Effort Sensors

Airflow and respiratory effort sensors can easily cause artifacts during polysomnography. An indication that airflow artifacts are present is when the nasal airflow is out of sync with the chest and abdominal airflow effort sensors. Respiratory effort recordings that are out of phase often indicate that one or more belts are too loose or too tight or have been dislodged by body movement. The sleep technologist must distinguish between recordings that indicate partial obstruction, which can result in out-of-phase respiratory effort recordings, and artifacts. Temperature-based and pressure-based sensors have different properties, so the technologist should be familiar with the properties and limitations of the sensors used when determining whether a recording represents an artifact.

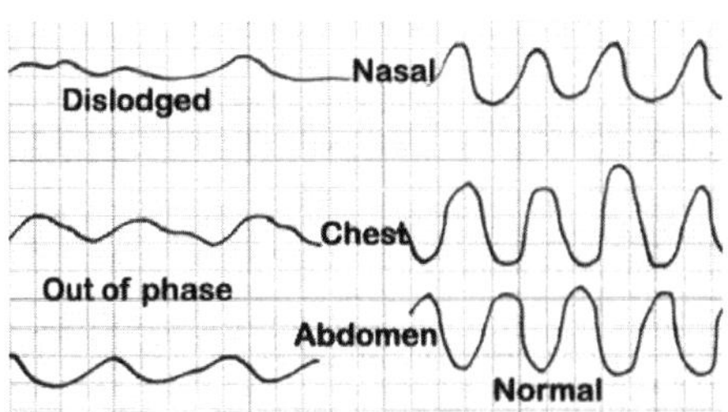

Movement Artifacts

Movement artifacts can cause distortion of all channels and may involve a number of other overlapping artifacts, such as electrode popping and muscle artifacts. Movement artifacts may be difficult to control and may interfere with recordings for patients who are extremely restless or move frequently during sleep. Often, excessive movement artifacts relate to improper application of electrodes or pulling on electrode wires as the patient turns. Securing the electrodes and making sure that the wires can accommodate turning and moving can reduce movement artifacts.

Muscle Artifacts

Muscle artifacts usually result from localized muscle activity near a reference or exploring electrode. Muscle artifacts can cause irregular distortion in multiple channels, such as the electroencephalogram and electrooculogram. Muscle artifacts can occur if a patient is extremely tense, so sometimes asking the patient to relax and slightly open the jaw can reduce artifacts. Artifacts may also relate to chewing movements or teeth grinding. In many cases, the electrodes should be re-referenced. The recording in the chin electromyogram is not considered an artifact because it is intended to measure muscle activity and normally increases with muscle tension or activity.

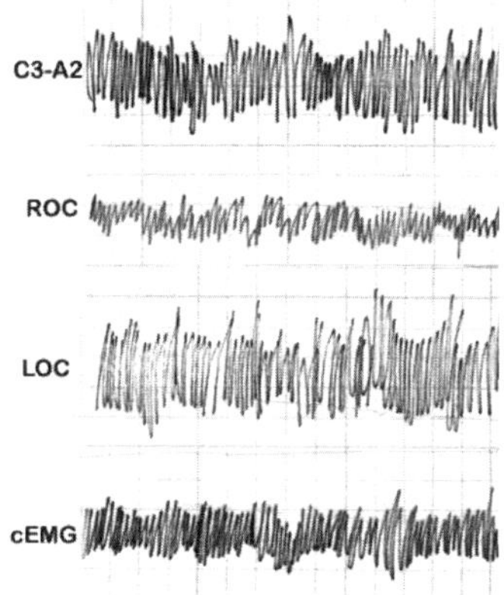

ECG Artifacts

Electrocardiogram (ECG) artifacts, recognizable by spikes that match the ECG recording in the electroencephalogram and electrooculogram channels, are common and not always avoidable, but they should not be prominent to the point that they obscure or confuse data. ECG artifacts are often more pronounced in obese patients, so reference electrodes should not be placed over soft fatty tissue. Double referencing the A1 and A2 reference electrodes can also minimize ECG artifacts; however, double referencing may cause increased interference from other types of artifacts, so double referencing should not be a routine procedure. ECG artifacts in the electromyogram channels usually indicate poor placement of electrodes or unequal impedances.

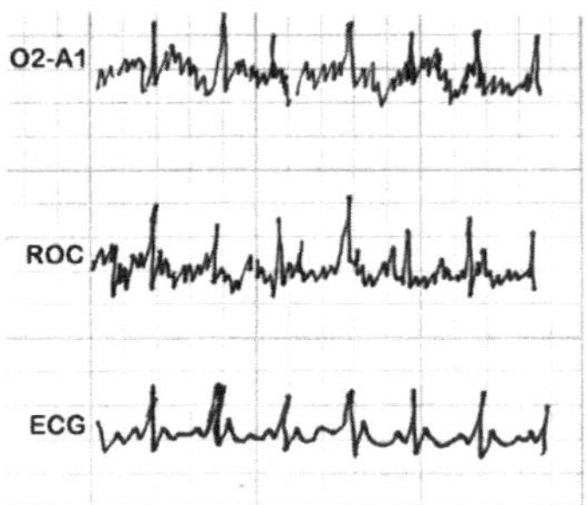

Slow-Frequency Artifacts

Slow-frequency artifacts can be related to perspiration, pressure on an electrode, or body movement.

Perspiration, the most common reason, results in chemical changes that cause a slow, frequently oscillating pattern that mirrors breathing patterns, often caused by small head movements with respirations. If caused by perspiration, lowering the temperature in the room by use of air conditioning or fans may help to resolve the problem. If caused by position, raising the low-frequency filter, changing the input derivation to the opposite side, or repositioning the patient may help. Careful and secure application of electrodes may decrease the incidence of slow-frequency artifacts.

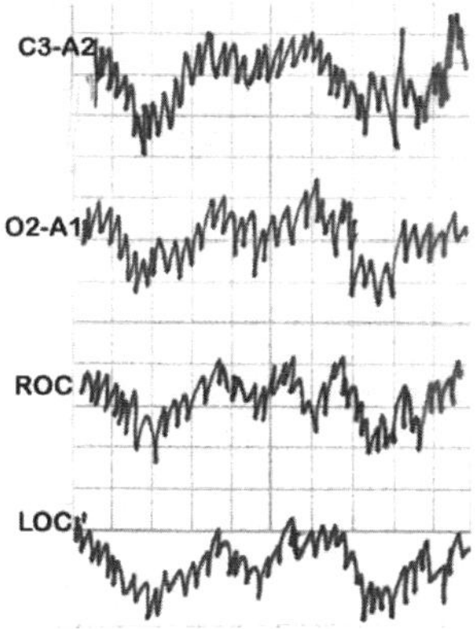

Oximetry Artifacts

Oximetry artifacts must be monitored carefully because interference may result in inaccurate readings that impact the study results. Inaccurate recordings may result from improper application of the oximeter, displacement (often related to movement), poor perfusion in distal extremities, motion artifacts, or inaccurate calibrations. Obesity may also interfere with oximetry recordings. The technologist should monitor the oximetry channel carefully and note irregular recordings, sudden variations, or abnormally low readings that do not correlate with other data. Oximetry artifacts must be tagged or removed from the recordings. Artifacts may be identified by noting changes in oxygen saturation in a consecutive series of sampling times. Pulse oximetry must always be correlated with other findings because pulse oximetry cannot identify sleep disorders that are unrelated to oxygen desaturation.

Parasomnias

Parasomnias	Polysomnogram
Confusional arousals	Shows alpha waves, repetitive periods of microsleep, or stage 1 non-REM sleep during arousal period
Enuresis	Typically normal
Exploding head syndrome	Shows sudden arousal during transition period between sleep and awakening, and electroencephalogram shows alpha and theta waves
Nightmares	Shows sudden arousal from REM sleep and abnormalities in REM sleep
REM sleep behavior disorder	Shows muscle activity during REM sleep
Sleep paralysis	Shows muscle atonia and alpha waves
Sleep-related eating	May show multiple arousals from stage 3 non-REM sleep and sometimes from REM sleep
Sleep-related groaning	Shows bradypnea and loud groaning in clusters, recurring several times during the night; otherwise normal
Sleep-related hallucinations	Shows onset usually during sleep-onset REM periods but also during non-REM sleep

Generating a Report

Formulas Related to Sleep Architecture

Apnea-hypopnea index	Number of apneas or hypopneas/hours of sleep (Number of apneas or hypopneas/minutes of sleep) x 60
Desaturation index	Number of desaturation events/hours of sleep (Number of desaturation events/minutes of sleep) x 60
Latency to persistent sleep	Number of epochs from lights out to first epoch of continuous sleep/2 (to provide time in minutes)
Latency to sleep stage	Number of epochs from sleep onset to onset of sleep stage/2 (to provide time in minutes)
Mean duration apnea or hypopnea	Total duration of apneas or hypopneas/number of apneas or hypopneas
Percent movement time	(Minutes of movement time/total sleep time) X 100
Respiratory disturbance index	Number of apneas + number of hypopneas + number of respiratory effort–related arousals (RERAs)/hours of sleep (Number of apneas + number of hypopneas + number of RERAs/minutes of sleep) x 60
Percent sleep efficiency	Total sleep time/total bed time x 100
Sleep onset	First of three consecutive epochs of stage 1 non-REM sleep
	Any stage 1 non-REM sleep
	Stage 1 non-REM sleep contiguous with stage 1 non-REM sleep
Sleep period time	Number of epochs/2
Percent sleep stage	(Minutes of sleep stage/total sleep time) X 100
Total recording time	Number of epochs from lights out to lights on/2 (to provide time in minutes)
Total sleep time	Addition of all sleep stages (stages 1, 2, and 3 non-REM and REM)
Total wake time	Wake before sleep + wake after sleep onset + wake after the sleep period

Components

The sleep study report is a record of the polysomnogram (PSG) and may vary, depending on the purpose of the study; however, it should be easily readable and understandable and should include both a clinical report and histograms that present a graphic representation of the results of the study. While computerized programs can quickly and easily produce a variety of different types of reports and graphs, the sleep technologist must evaluate all aspects of the PSG and score events to corroborate computer-generated reports. The clinical report should include: sleep architecture, sleep stages, apnea events, hypopnea events, respiratory events, body positions (supine and non-supine), respiratory events with arousals, periodic leg movements and sleep stages with and without arousals, spontaneous arousals, oxygen saturation, and pressure level analysis with calibrations for continuous positive airway pressure and bilevel positive airway pressure. The identifiers on the sleep study report should include the following:

- Patient's name, identification number, age, and gender
- Test date
- Relevant history and medications
- Height and weight
- Reason for referral

Sleep Parameters, Stages, and Arousals

Sleep parameters must be totaled and summarized in the sleep study report. These parameters include the following:

- Study start time, study end time, and total study time
- Lights off time and lights on time
- Sleep period time in minutes, hours, and number of epochs
- Total sleep time (TST) in minutes, hours, and number of epochs
- Sleep onset time in minutes
- Sleep efficiency as a percentage of TST
- Latency to stage 1 non-REM in minutes
- REM sleep latency in minutes.

Stages of sleep (stages 1, 2, and 3 non-REM, REM, W) should be reported in minutes, percentage of TST, and minutes of latencies.

Arousals should be reported as a total number, index number, and numbers occurring in REM sleep and in non-REM sleep for all different types and associations. Specific types of arousal situations should include those associated with desaturations, periodic leg movements, obstructive sleep apnea, respiratory events, mixed apneas, central apnea, hypopneas, and snoring.

Leg Movements, Respiratory Events, and Comments

Leg movements should be classified according to type: total periodic movements, periodic movements with arousal, total isolated movements, and total isolated movements with arousal. Numbers should be indicated for movements occurring in REM sleep, non-REM sleep, totals, and index.

Respiratory events should be classified as central apneas, mixed apneas, obstructive events, and hypopneas with the numbers reported for non-REM sleep, REM sleep, and totals. Additional information can include mean duration, minimum duration, and maximum duration (in minutes) for each during non-REM and REM sleep.

Comments by the technologist can contain valuable information regarding the patient's emotional and physical status. The technologist should report visual or audible findings, such as snoring, unusual motor activity, or parasomnias. The technologist should make note of information that may not be evident from the recordings but can impact the diagnosis or treatment.

Data Storage

Data storage of the patient's raw data and reports, including diagnoses and treatments, is mandated by the American Academy of Sleep Medicine. Data must be saved in such a way that access is limited to authorized personnel only because of regulations related to privacy and confidentiality. Digital recordings may be stored electronically with backup so that data are not lost. Paper recordings may be stored in patient charts. Digital files may vary in size from 50–150 megabytes, which can usually be stored on the individual computer system, but eventually the files need to be archived to make room for other recordings. This may mean transferring the information to an external hard drive, a recordable device (CD or DVD), or an optical disc. Data may also be transferred to a large central database. Policies and procedures must be in place regarding data storage.

Archiving Polysomnogram Reports

Archiving polysomnogram reports, like all medical data, can be achieved by a number of methods, but in all cases the data must be stored in secure facilities or in secure electronic storage for a number of years.

- Storing paper documents: Data are difficult to retrieve, and storage is space intensive.
- Creating back-up tapes: This requires a storage area and often temperature control as tapes may degrade over time.
- WORM (write once/read many) technology: This is available as optical or magnetic discs and tapes. It provides data storage that cannot be edited, altered, or recorded over, so it meets legal requirements for data storage; however, the data must be password protected as it may be accessed easily over a network.
- Disc (CD/DVD) storage. Discs can be corrupted or demagnetized.
- "Cloud" storage: Archives are saved electronically outside the facility, by companies that specialize in providing secure storage for data.

Understanding Sleep Disorders

PROCEDURE ORDERS

Procedure orders are usually generated by the attending physician and are explicit about the type of testing, including any special orders to accommodate special needs, such as for the patient with dementia or diabetes; procedure orders must be signed and dated. Orders include any routine medications the patient takes before or during the test. Since most states do not allow sleep technicians to administer medications, medications are either self-administered, or other licensed staff is available to administer them. Technicians must be aware of the medications taken by the patient in the event the patient terminates the testing and leaves the facility, which may put the patient or others in danger, if, for example, the patient has taken sleeping medication. The procedure orders are checked in relation to the patient questionnaire to resolve any discrepancies, and the physician is contacted if necessary.

HISTORY AND PHYSICAL

The history and physical is reviewed by the technician before the first meeting with the patient, if possible, as this information can guide the initial assessment as well as the evaluation during and after the testing.

Sleep disorders	Obstructive/central sleep apnea, narcolepsy, circadian rhythm disorders, restless legs syndrome, periodic leg movement, parasomnias, and insomnia
Respiratory disorders	Chronic obstructive pulmonary disease, cystic fibrosis, restrictive lung diseases, and asthma
Neuromuscular diseases	Multiple sclerosis, amyotrophic lateral sclerosis, myasthenia gravis, poliomyelitis, and myotonic dystrophy
Spinal cord injury	Bilateral diaphragmatic paralysis
Gastrointestinal disorders	Gastroesophageal reflux disease and functional bowel disorders
Endocrine disorders	Hypothyroidism, acromegaly, Cushing's syndrome, Addison's disease, diabetes mellitus, and diabetes insipidus.
Rheumatologic disorders	Pain syndromes and fibromyalgia
Kidney/urinary disorders	End-stage renal disease and urinary frequency
Infectious diseases	HIV/AIDS, Lyme disease, and human African trypanosomiasis
Cardiovascular disorders	Heart block, dysrhythmias, congestive heart failure, coronary artery disease, and atrial fibrillation
Psychiatric disorders	Bipolar disorder, depression, post-traumatic stress disorder, and schizophrenia

PRIMARY INSOMNIA

Primary insomnia is difficulty falling asleep, staying asleep, a combination of both, or having non-refreshing sleep for at least 1 month, with onset usually after a stressful episode, resulting in impairment of work, study, and social activities. Individuals may have anxiety and functional impairment and are at risk for mood disorders. Polysomnography may show that continuity of sleep is interrupted with increased alpha and beta waves during sleep, although people usually are not sleepy in the daytime but may appear lethargic. They may exhibit variability in sleeping patterns from one night to another. They typically experience increased stage 1 and decreased stages 2 and 3 sleep. They may also complain of stress-related disorders, such as muscle tension and headaches, and may exhibit increased reactions to stress and increased metabolic rate. Individuals sometimes report better sleep in the polysomnography lab than at home. Insomnia is a common problem occurring in up to 35% of adults at some time with chronic insomnia in 10%–15%. Insomnia may be precipitated by physical conditions, such as heart disease, gastroesophageal reflux disease, urinary incontinence, or psychiatric disorders. Insomnia is common with depression and bipolar disorder.

Chronic Insomnia

Chronic insomnia occurs over prolonged periods of time and has several forms.

Psychological	This is a self-perpetuating form in which anxiety about the inability to sleep interferes with sleeping. Polysomnography shows increased wakefulness, increased sleep latency, and decreased sleep efficiency.
Sleep-state misperception	Polysomnography shows normal sleep, but the patient reports reduced or no sleep and often does not believe contrary lab results.
Hypnotic dependent sleep disorder	The patient develops a tolerance to hypnotics, requiring ever increasing doses, and is unable to sleep without medication. Withdrawal results in insomnia, nervousness, and agitation.
Fatal familial insomnia	This is a fatal neurologic disorder in which the patient has difficulty falling asleep, progressing to an inability to sleep. A desynchronized electroencephalogram and an absence of slow-wave sleep characterize this disorder.

Hypersomnia

Hypersomnia is characterized by increased sleepiness and prolonged nocturnal sleep (8–12 hours) and daytime sleepiness (characterized by intentional or non-intentional napping) on a daily basis for at least a month with difficulty awakening, resulting in social, occupational, and other impairment. Intentional naps usually last an hour or more and non-intentional napping occurs during times of low stimulation, such as while watching television or driving. Nocturnal polysomnography shows normal to prolonged sleep and sleep continuity with normal REM and non-REM periods. The multiple sleep latency test shows excess sleepiness during the daytime with mean sleep latency of 5–10 minutes. Onset is usually between the ages of 15 and 30 years with symptoms worsening over time and eventually stabilizing. The recurrent form lasts for periods of at least 3 days and occurs several times yearly for 2 years or more.

Narcolepsy

Narcolepsy is characterized by repeated periods of falling asleep during waking hours daily for at least 3 months. Onset is often during childhood or adolescence and is rare after 40 years of age. Onset is often preceded by an acute psychological stressor or disruption of the sleep-wake schedule. Narcolepsy can include cataplexy (sudden loss of muscle tone) or recurrent rapid eye movement during the transition period between wakefulness and sleep, causing voluntary muscle paralysis and hallucinations. Narcolepsy is a rare disorder occurring in only 0.02%–0.16% of adults. The multiple sleep latency test shows mean sleep latency of less than 5 minutes and REM sleep during two or more of five naps. Nocturnal polysomnography shows sleep latencies of less than 10 minutes and sleep-onset REM sleep with increased eye movement during REM periods. Episodes of sleep apnea and periodic limb movement may be evident.

Obstructive Sleep Apnea

Obstructive sleep apnea results from the passive collapse of the pharynx during sleep, often associated with a narrow or restricted upper airway from micrognathia, obesity, or enlarged tonsils. It is most common in middle-aged, overweight men and is exacerbated by drinking alcohol or ingesting sedative drugs before sleeping. Symptoms include daytime somnolence, headache, cognitive impairment, depression, personality changes, recent increase in weight, and impotence. Patients often snore loudly with cycles of breath cessation caused by apneic periods up to 60 seconds, occurring at least 30 times a night despite continued chest wall and abdominal movements, indicating an automatic attempt to breathe. Electrocardiographic changes may indicate bradydysrhythmia during apnea and tachydysrhythmia when breathing resumes. Nocturnal polysomnography shows apneic periods for over 10 seconds (usually 20–40 seconds). There may be hypopnea with reduction of airflow. Both apneic and hypopneic periods result in reduced oxyhemoglobin saturation. If this condition is severe, hypoxemia or hypercarbia may persist during waking hours.

Central Sleep Apnea and Central Alveolar Hypoventilation Syndrome

Central sleep apnea involves apneic and hypopneic episodes without obstruction and usually results from cardiac or neurological disorders that cause impairment of ventilation. Snoring is usually mild, and individuals may complain of insomnia because they awaken frequently. Chest wall and abdominal movements do not occur during apneic periods with this breathing-related sleep disorder. Cheyne-Stokes respirations may be present (apnea, 10–60 seconds of hyperventilation, followed by another period of apnea). Nocturnal polysomnography shows decreased respiratory effort associated with decreased oxygen saturation.

Central alveolar hypoventilation syndrome results from impaired ventilatory control, characterized by low arterial oxygen levels and hypoventilation without apnea or hypopnea. Hypoventilation periods may persist for several minutes with sustained arterial oxygen desaturation and increased levels of carbon dioxide. This condition is often associated with obesity. Individuals may complain of feeling excessively sleepy or having insomnia. If this condition is severe, hypoxemia or hypercarbia may persist during waking hours.

Restless Legs Syndrome and Periodic Leg Movements of Sleep

Restless legs syndrome (RLS) is characterized by pain and paresthesia in the legs at rest, especially in the evening and at night when trying to sleep. Some people also have periodic jerking of limbs. Moving the legs relieves leg discomfort, but this often results in difficulty sleeping and resultant exhaustion during the daytime, so patients may complain of insomnia. Neurological examination is typically normal, but a family history of RLS is common. Some people have relief of symptoms if they reduce caffeine, alcohol, and tobacco use. RLS does not require polysomnography because it is an awake disorder that interferes with sleep rather than a direct sleep disorder. RLS can be evaluated with the suggested immobilization test to diagnose periodic limb movement of wakefulness (PLMW). RLS is diagnosed with more than 40 PLMW an hour.

Periodic leg movements of sleep (PLMS) are similar but occur during sleep and are often associated with RLS (occurring in about 80% of patients with RLS) with five or more PLMS usually within the first half of the night. PLMS is common in other patients and may be noted on anterior tibialis electromyogram, but these movements may not be clinically relevant.

Circadian Rhythm Sleep Disorder Both Delayed and Advanced Sleep Phase Types

Circadian rhythm sleep disorder relates to altered functioning of the circadian sleep–wake system or imposed mismatch between the patient's natural sleep–wake system and required sleep–wake system (common in shift workers). Subtypes include:

- Delayed sleep phase: Patients tend to fall asleep late at night and cannot initiate sleep earlier, so they may have much difficulty awakening at required times, requiring multiple alarms to awaken. However, they may sleep adequately if left to their own schedules, such as on nonworking days. When patients are sleeping at preferred times, polysomnography is essentially normal, but at other times, patients exhibit delay in sleep-onset, short duration of sleep, and short periods of REM sleep.
- Advanced sleep phase: The opposite of delayed sleep phase, patients fall asleep in the early evening and awaken in the early hours of the morning. Testing is normal if sleeping at preferred times, but sleep deprivation may occur if patients stay awake in the evening for social or other reasons.

Circadian Rhythm Sleep Disorder from Jet Leg, Shift Work, and Unspecified

Circadian rhythm sleep disorder subtypes include the following:

- Jet lag: Patients travel to different time zones and cannot adapt their sleep–wake cycle so they may experience fatigue, disorientation, and lack of adequate sleep with a degree of symptoms related to the number of time zones. West-to-east travel is usually more poorly tolerated than east-to-west travel.
- Shift work: While the patient's sleep cycle is normal, work requirements disrupt this cycle, forcing the person to sleep outside the cycle, often resulting in shorter periods of sleep and chronic fatigue. Polysomnography shows normal or short sleep latency and reduced duration of sleep and may display an increased disturbance of sleep. Patients may also have a reduction in stages 1 and 3 non-REM and REM sleep. Patients typically exhibit high degrees of sleepiness on the multiple sleep latency test.
- Unspecified/advanced delay: The cycles of these patients tend to increase in delay so that sleeping patterns change over time with the patient falling asleep at increasingly later hours.

Nightmare Disorder

Nightmare disorder, sometimes associated with post-traumatic stress disorder (PTSD), describes repeated nightmares that cause the patient to awaken fully alert, interrupting the normal sleep cycle. Nightmares occur during REM sleep and tend to occur in the second half of the night when REM periods are longer. The patient may suffer from fatigue from lack of sleep caused by frequent awakening or may avoid sleeping because of fear of the nightmares. Because muscle tone is lost during REM sleep, nightmare disorder is not usually accompanied by talking, screaming, or hitting, but these may occur at the end of the nightmare in some individuals, especially those with PTSD. Polysomnography shows sudden awakening from REM sleep with reports of nightmares, typically in the second half of the night after REM periods lasting more than 10 minutes. Electrooculogram may show increased eye movements. Electrocardiogram shows increased heart rate, and respiratory sensors show increased respiratory rate.

Sleep Terror Disorder

Sleep terror disorder (night terrors) is awakening abruptly, primarily during the first third of the night. It occurs in children between the ages of 4 and 12 and usually resolves by adolescence. In adults, onset is usually between the ages of 20 and 30. Typically, the person sits up in bed and screams or cries and may flail about or fight against being touched but cannot be easily awakened. The episodes, lasting 1 to 10 minutes, include an autonomic response with increased heart rate, tachypnea, flushing, sweating, increased muscle tone, and pupil dilation. Once awakened, the person usually does not recall the dream but feels frightened. The person falls quickly back to sleep and has no memory of the episode on awakening in the morning. Sleep terror disorder may be associated with sleepwalking. Polysomnography shows onset during non-REM sleep with delta waves on the electroencephalogram, although theta or alpha activity may be evident during the episode, suggesting partial arousal. The electrocardiogram shows a heart rate up to 120 beats/minute. The electromyogram shows increased activity.

Sleepwalking Disorder

Sleepwalking disorder (somnambulism) is characterized by motor activity during sleep, including sitting up, picking at bedding, talking, walking, running, operating machinery, and eating. During the episode, the patient may respond verbally to others, but speech may not be clear because of reduced alertness. The patient's eyes are usually open. Patients may also urinate in inappropriate places. Typically, the patient does not awaken easily and is confused if awakened and has little or no memory of the episode. Nocturnal polysomnography and audiovisual monitoring show motor activity. Onset is usually during stage 3 non-REM sleep for children, although adults may have onset during stage 2 non-REM sleep, within the first few hours of sleep. The electroencephalogram (EEG) shows high-voltage delta waves before and during the episode and sometimes alpha waves at onset, but artifacts caused by motor activity may obscure EEG activity. The electrocardiogram shows increased heart rate, and respiratory sensors show increased respirations. Patients may have increased transitions from stage 3 non-REM sleep and increased episodes of awakening during non-REM sleep.

Parasomnias

Parasomnias, physical phenomena associated with sleep, comprise a number of different disorders of arousal, occurring primarily during stage 3 non-REM sleep, in the first third of the night and are most common during childhood.

Confusional arousals	The patient, usually a child, is confused and disoriented on arousal for minutes or hours.
Enuresis	Enuresis is repeated, involuntary, urinary incontinence in children old enough to have bladder control, usually about 5–6 years old. Enuresis is most common in the first third of the night with the child awakening after urinating. There are three types: Primary: The child has never been dry at night, and incontinence is associated with delay in maturation and small functional bladder rather than stress or psychiatric disorders. Intermittent: The child stays dry part of the time with episodes of incontinence at night. Secondary: The child has had long periods (6–12 months) of staying dry.
Exploding head syndrome	Upon awakening, the patient perceives a sudden (imaginary) noise or explosion, sometimes accompanied by a flash of light, jerking, and fright.
Nightmares	Frightening dreams occur during REM sleep in the latter part of the night.

REM sleep behavior disorder	During REM sleep, periods of muscle activity occur in which the patient may act out motor activities of the dream, such as flailing arms, kicking, hitting, running, and jumping out of bed. Typically, the patient's eyes are closed during the episode, which is most common in men 60–70 years of age.
Sleep paralysis	Muscle atonia occurs during onset of sleep (hypnagogic) or on waking (hypnopompic), most often during adolescence. The patient can see and breathe but is not able to move for periods of seconds to minutes.
Sleep-related eating	The patient eats during the night and has no recollection of doing so. This is distinct from night eating syndrome in which the patient is aware of eating but unable to go back to sleep without eating. Some sleeping medications may precipitate sleep-related eating. Sleep-related eating carries the risk of choking or aspiration.
Sleep-related groaning	Sleep-related groaning (catathrenia) occurs during exhalation, primarily during REM sleep. The respirations become slow, and the groaning exhalation may persist for 30–40 seconds, usually concluding with a grunting or sighing sound.
Sleep-related hallucinations	Visual, auditory, or tactile hallucinations occur during onset of sleep (hypnagogic) or on waking (hypnopompic), sometimes associated with sleep paralysis. Images tend to be stationary and disappear if the light is switched on.

Substance-Induced Sleep Disorder

Substance-induced sleep disorder can be caused by intoxication and withdrawal from alcohol as well as many other different drugs. Subtypes include insomnia, hypersomnia, parasomnia, and mixed.

Drug	Disorder	Characteristics
Alcohol intoxication	Insomnia	Sedation occurs during acute intoxications with increased sleeping and decreased wakefulness for 3–4 hours with increased non-REM stages 3 and 4 sleep and reduced REM sleep. After this period, the patient experiences decreased stage 3 non-REM sleep, increased wakefulness, and increased REM sleep with restlessness and sometimes vivid dreams.
Alcohol withdrawal	Insomnia	Gross disturbance of sleep with an increase in the amount of REM sleep, often with vivid dreams. After withdrawal, insomnia with a light restless sleep may persist for weeks to years with a deficit in slow-wave sleep.
Amphetamines/ related drugs: intoxication	Insomnia	Typically, total sleep is reduced with increased sleep latency and sleep disturbance. EMG shows increased muscular activity. REM sleep and slow-wave sleep decrease.
Amphetamines/ related drugs: withdrawal	Hypersomnia	Prolonged sleeping during the night. REM and slow-wave sleep may increase above baseline. MSLT shows increased sleepiness during the daytime as well.

Drug	Disorder	Characteristics
Caffeine use	Insomnia	Increased wakefulness and decreased sleep are dose dependent. Polysomnography shows increased sleep latency and wakefulness and decreased slow-wave sleep.
Caffeine withdrawal	Hypersomnia	Increased sleeping and daytime sleepiness are common.
Cocaine intoxication	Insomnia	Sleep is severely compromised, and the patient may sleep only for short, disrupted periods.
Cocaine withdrawal	Hypersomnia	Sleep is markedly prolonged.
Opioid use (chronic)	Insomnia	While acute use of opioids may result in increased sleepiness with reduced REM sleep, chronic use may cause insomnia with increased wakefulness and decreased sleep time.
Opioid withdrawal	Hypersomnia	Sleep is prolonged.
Sedative/ hypnotic intoxication	Hypersomnia	Initial sedative effects result in an increase in sleepiness, decreased wakefulness, and a decrease in REM sleep with an increase in sleep-spindle activity.
Sedative/ hypnotic chronic use/withdrawal	Mixed insomnia and hypersomnia	As the patient develops a tolerance for the drug, sedative effects decrease, and insomnia occurs. If the patient increases the dose of medication to compensate, then hypersomnia recurs. Withdrawal often results in insomnia with a decrease in sleep duration and an increased disruption of sleep and REM sleep rebound as well as anxiety, tremors, and ataxia.
Antiarrhythmics (quinidine, procainamide)	Insomnia	These drugs may cause disruption of sleep during the night and increased sleepiness in the waking hours.
Antihistamines (diphenhydramine, Benadryl)	Hypersomnia	Some drugs may produce a sedative effect, causing increased sleeping during the night and increased sleepiness during the daytime.
β-Blockers	Insomnia	β-Blockers decrease sleep, increase disruption of sleep, and increase nightmares.
Bronchodilators (theophylline)	Insomnia	High doses of some bronchodilators may cause nervousness, muscle cramping, twitching, and sleep disruption.
Corticosteroids	Insomnia	Steroids may markedly decrease sleep time and increase time needed to fall asleep as well as cause fatigue and jitters during the day.
Diuretics	Insomnia	Decreasing potassium levels may cause leg cramps that interfere with sleeping, and the increase in urinary output may cause nocturia, interrupting sleep.
Nicotine patches	Insomnia	Patches may interfere with falling asleep and duration of sleep and cause vivid dreams or nightmares.

Drug	Disorder	Characteristics
Selective serotonin reuptake inhibitors (SSRIs)	Insomnia	Some individuals experience sleep disruption and sleepiness during waking hours when taking SSRIs.
Thyroid hormone (Synthroid)	Insomnia	High doses of thyroid hormone may cause nervousness, tremors, heart palpitations, and disruption of sleep.

Abbreviations: EMG = electromyogram; and MSLT = multiple sleep latency test.

Alzheimer's Disease

Alzheimer's disease and other causes of dementia result in behavior that can contribute to sleep problems. Dementia may interfere with sleep, and patients may have undiagnosed and untreated obstructive sleep apnea or other sleep disorders.

Sundowners: Patients often have disruption of the sleep–wake cycle, and sundowner's syndrome, in which the person becomes increasingly agitated and restless in the evening, is common as dementia advances. The patient may get up to urinate and forget to return to bed, disrupting the sleep–wake cycle. Others may nap frequently during the daytime, making them less tired at night.

Wandering: Patients may become confused and begin to wander during the night or day and may become frightened and hide, compounding the problem. It is not clear why patients wander, but perhaps there is a physical need, such as the need to drink or urinate, that prompts them to get up and start walking. In some cases, they may just be walking and get lost.

Patients' Identification and Informed Consent

Patients' identification is checked by the sleep technologist, following protocol established by the facility, and the records are reviewed carefully to ensure that the correct patient identifier is on all paper and computer records.

Informed consent is provided by patients or family for all treatments the patient receives. This includes a thorough explanation of all procedures and treatments with their associated risks. Patients or family are apprised of all options and allowed input on the types of treatment. Patients or family are apprised of all reasonable risks and any complications that might be life-threatening or increase morbidity. The American Medical Association has established guidelines for informed consent:

- Explanation of diagnosis
- Nature and reason for treatment or procedure
- Risks and benefits
- Alternative options (regardless of cost or insurance coverage)
- Risks and benefits of alternative options
- Risks and benefits of not having a treatment or procedure
- Providing informed consent (a requirement of all states)

Pediatrics

Informed consent for medical treatments and testing cannot be provided by children younger than 18 years of age (minors), unless they are legally emancipated, until they reach the age of majority, except for certain treatments or testing approved by law, such as for birth control, abortion, and

HIV testing; however, even laws concerning these situations vary from state to state, with some requiring parental notification. However, children must be included in discussions about treatment options and testing in accordance with their age and level of understanding. Because children do not always appreciate cause and effect relationships, the law allows the parents to override decisions of the child and teenager, but forcing a child to have treatment or testing puts the child in a poor emotional state and is cause for ethical concern. Therefore, the sleep technologist should work with both the parents and the child, explaining the benefits and disadvantages of testing, to bring about agreement or assent on the part of the child. This is especially important for adolescents, who are seeking autonomy.

Pre-Sleep Interview

Pre-sleep interviews are conducted by sleep technicians, who ask questions to clarify information and make careful observations of the patient during the interview, noting the patient's appearance; level of alertness; readiness to learn or obstacles to learning (e.g., language differences, dementia); mental age; and physical limitations, such as hearing impairment or paralysis. The patient's emotional state is assessed as well as any concerns the patient may have about the testing. For example, patients with post-traumatic stress disorder may react violently if awakened abruptly during the night, so the sleep technician must learn about the patient's preferred method of being aroused before testing. Patients with claustrophobia may not be able to tolerate a facemask. The technologist notes information gained from the interview on the patient's record. In most sleep centers, a general questionnaire, including a history and a list of medications, is completed before the presleep questionnaire. The general questionnaire is compared with the physician's history and physical, and any additions or discrepancies are noted.

Pre-Sleep Questionnaire

Pre-sleep questionnaires are usually standardized forms that review issues related to sleep, but the technologist asks additional questions for clarification as needed. The questionnaire helps to determine if the patient's preceding 24 hours were normal for that individual. Topics covered include the following:

Sleep preparation	Activities done before bedtime, such as showering, exercising, watching television, or reading in bed
Sleep patterns	Usual time to bed, time to rise, and time needed to fall asleep
Sleep position	Side lying, supine, prone, and number of pillows
Sleep problems	Restlessness, restless legs, insomnia, snoring, gasping, choking, or apneic periods
Sleep arrangement	Sleeps alone, has bed partner, or sleeps with animals on bed
Sleep aids	Sleeping medications, music, television, or reading
Habits	Smoking, drinking, including the type, amount, and time used within 24 hours of testing
Nocturia	Frequency of using the bathroom during the night
Other physical complaints	Dry mouth on arising, nasal congestion, or headaches in the morning
Daytime patterns	Sleepiness in the morning, tiredness through day, falling asleep inappropriately, needing naps, and duration and frequency of naps
Medications	All medications taken within 24 hours of testing

Sleep Diaries

Sleep diaries are invaluable to the patients' assessment. The patient keeps a record of sleep habits for a 2-week period preceding the test. The sleep diary generally has two components:

- Before sleep: Patient assesses mood with a 1–5 scale that ranges from bad mood to excellent mood, notes any medications taken (especially sleeping medications) and the time the lights are turned off.
- Upon awakening: Patient estimates the approximate time to onset of sleep and the number of arousals during the night and the time of awakening. The patient assesses mood with a 1–5 scale.

Patient's perceptions about the time needed to fall asleep and the number of awakenings that occur during the night may be considerably at odds with the findings during the polysomnogram. The patient may simply be mistaken, or the patient's experience in the sleep center is different. For example, some people find it very difficult to sleep during the test or may arouse more easily in a strange environment.

Bed-Partner Questionnaires

Bed-partner questionnaires are filled out by the patient's bed partner (or in some cases a roommate or parent) with the patient's permission. The partner is often aware of snoring or periods of apnea even though the patient is not. A typical questionnaire includes the following information:

- Patient and reporter's names
- Frequency with which the reporter has observed the patient sleeping
- Positions in which the patient typically sleeps (back, stomach, right side, left side) and an estimate of the percentage of the night in each position
- Descriptions of sleep behaviors (usually with a checklist):
  - Type of snoring: light, loud, or snorting
  - Respiratory changes: choking or pauses
  - Extremities: twitching or jerking
  - Seizure-like activity: rigidity or shaking
  - Mouth activity: teeth grinding
  - Abnormal sleep behavior: sleep walking, talking, crying, sitting up, banging head, or rocking
  - Awakening behavior: alert, lethargic, or complaining of pain

Morning/Evening Questionnaires

Morning/evening questionnaires ask nineteen questions about time preferences, providing a range of answers that determines if the person is a morning, evening, or neutral person. (In 1976, Horne and Ostberg studied sleep patterns and classified people as "morning" or "evening" people, depending on their preferences for sleeping and arising and level of alertness.) Questions include:

- The time of day the patient would get up and go to bed if free to decide
- The degree of dependency on an alarm clock to awaken at the normally scheduled time
- The ease of getting up in the morning
- The patient's feelings and appetite in the half hour after awakening

The time of day the patient gets up on days with no obligations in relation to normal time to arise; The ease with which the patient could engage in sports activities between 7 and 8 am or 10 and 11 pm; The time of day at which the patient feels tired enough to fall asleep; The 2 hours during the day the patient would prefer to study for an exam; How the patient feels in the morning after going to sleep at 11 pm; The time the patient would arise after going to bed several hours late; when the patient would sleep if having to stand guard from 4–6 am; The 2 hours during the day the patient would prefer to exercise; The 5 consecutive hours during the day the patient would prefer to work; The hour the patient feels the best

Whether the patient considers him- or herself a morning or evening person

Registered Sleep Technologist Practice Test

Want to take this practice test in an online interactive format?
Check out the online resources page, which includes interactive practice questions and much more: **mometrix.com/resources719/regsleeptech**

1. Which of the following is characteristic of sleep during the second trimester of pregnancy?

a. Total sleep time (TST) decreases to pre-pregnancy levels
b. Slow-wave sleep (SWS) decreases
c. REM sleep decreases
d. Shortness of breath decreases

2. The amount of blood that is pumped through the ventricles is known as

a. cardiac output
b. pulmonary vascular resistance
c. stroke volume
d. cardiac index

3. Twitching movements of the fingers, toes, and mouth that may occur during stage W, non-REM, and REM sleep are known as

a. bruxism
b. excessive fragmentary myoclonus(EFM)
c. REM sleep behavior disorder (RBD)
d. rhythmic movement disorder(RMD)

4. What is the purpose of the American Sleep Apnea Association's A.W.A.K.E. program?

a. To provide specialized training to future sleep technologists
b. To provide education, guidance, and ongoing support for sleep apnea
c. To diagnose sleep apnea
d. To fit sleep apnea patients with continuous positive airway pressure masks

5. The cEMG provides information on all of the following EXCEPT

a. snoring
b. teeth grinding
c. electrical activity within the brain
d. muscle tone of the chin muscles

6. Which of the following constitutes good sleep hygiene?

a. Drinking alcohol before going to bed
b. Watching TV in bed right before trying to go to sleep
c. Getting up to do something relaxing after 20 minutes in bed
d. Taking naps during the day

7. Atrial fibrillation is characterized by all of the following EXCEPT

a. an atrial rate of 120-200 beats/min and a ventricular rate of 300-600 beats/min
b. normal shape and duration of the QRS complex
c. the presence of fibrillatory (F) waves instead of P waves
d. a highly variable P:QRS ratio

8. In generalized anxiety disorder, polysomnography is characterized by which of the following?

a. Increased stage 1 non-REM sleep
b. Increased REM density
c. Quick onset of sleep
d. All of the above

9. Which of the following brain structures is involved in autonomic functions, homeostasis, endocrine processes, emotions, and the regulation of sleep?

a. Hypothalamus
b. Mamillary bodies
c. Hippocampus
d. Posterior pituitary gland

10. For home treatment with positive airway pressure, proper humidifier care includes

a. using only tap water for humidification
b. emptying the water reservoir once per week
c. washing the reservoir with bleach
d. rinsing and air-drying the reservoir

11. Morning/evening questionnaires ask the patient to indicate which of the following?

a. How the patient feels in the morning after going to sleep at 9 PM
b. The five consecutive hours during the day that the patient would prefer to work
c. The patient's appetite two hours after awakening
d. All of the above

12. Which of the following is FALSE with regard to hematocrit?

a. A decrease in hematocrit can be indicative of anemia
b. It measures the percentage of packed white blood cells in 100 mL of blood
c. An increase in hematocrit can be indicative of dehydration
d. Normal hematocrit values for men are 42%–52%

13. One criterion for scoring pediatric obstructive sleep apnea is that, compared to baseline, there is a 90% or greater decrease in amplitude for at least what percentage of events?

a. 25%
b. 50%
c. 80%
d. 90%

14. Sudden, involuntary, abnormal electrical disturbances in the brain that can manifest as alterations of consciousness, convulsions, and loss of consciousness are known as

a. generalized tonic-clonic seizures
b. primary generalized myoclonic epilepsy
c. amyotrophic lateral sclerosis
d. West syndrome

15. A type 2 sleep study must include all of the following EXCEPT

a. EEG channel
b. EOG channel
c. pulse oximetry
d. testing at a sleep center

16. What is the range of normal scores on the Fatigue Severity Scale?

a. 5-15
b. 5-20
c. 9-25
d. 9-35

17. Which of the following is NOT part of scoring pediatric obstructive sleep apneas?

a. A duration of two or more missed respirations (or duration of two respirations based on baseline recordings)
b. Inspiratory effort that continues or increases throughout the apneic period
c. Missed respirations associated with arousal, awakening, or desaturation of 3% or more
d. A 90% or more decrease in amplitude for 90% or more of events, compared to baseline

18. Ketonuria, Kussmaul respirations, hyperglycemia, and fluid imbalance are characteristic of

a. stroke
b. myocardial infarction(MI)
c. acute asthma attack
d. diabetic ketoacidosis(DKA)

19. What is the highest grade level at which patient education materials and consent forms for polysomnography should be written?

a. 2nd to 4th grade
b. 3rd to 4th grade
c. 4th to 6th grade
d. 6th to 8th grade

20. In a patient with pseudohypertrophic Duchenne muscular dystrophy, which of the following is NOT a typical sleep-related problem?

a. Hypercapnia and oxygen desaturation during sleep
b. Decrease in vital capacity to less than 2 L
c. Central sleep apnea
d. Increasing sleep disruption

21. Which type of waves have a frequency of 13–35 Hz, an amplitude of less than 30 µV, and are present during normal wakefulness when the patient is alert?

a. Delta waves
b. Beta waves
c. Vertex waves
d. Theta waves

22. During polysomnography, which of the following can be created by skin irritation, such as a rash?

a. High-frequency artifacts
b. Spike in EEG
c. High impedance
d. Slow waves

23. Pulse oximetry measures

a. arterial oxygen saturation (SpO_2)
b. electrical activity in the leg muscles
c. vertical and horizontal eye movements
d. the degree and duration of snoring

24. When periodic limb movements of sleep are scored as events, which of the following is FALSE?

a. An event ranges in duration from 0.5–10 seconds, with an EMG amplitude of 8 µV or more
b. Timing of the event begins at the point of an 8-µV increase on EMG
c. Timing of the event ends with a period, lasting 0.5 seconds or longer, during which EMG does not rise more than 2 µV
d. An event requires four or more consecutive leg movements, with the interval between movements ranging from 5-90 seconds

25. Which of the following is NOT a way to decrease the amount of condensation in humidifier tubing?

a. Using heated tubing
b. Reducing the level of humidification
c. Insulating the tubing
d. Decreasing room temperature at night

26. Which of the following is true with regard to electrode impedances?

a. Electrodes should be tested together in groups of three
b. When there is a difference in impedance between electrodes, the number of artifacts is reduced
c. Impedance levels for each individual electrode should be less than or equal to 5 kΩ
d. The technologist should verify the electrode impedances before calibrating the machine

27. Which of the following is FALSE with regard to liquid oxygen?

a. It is stored at -183°C in special cryogenic containers
b. It is maintained at 18 psi
c. As the tanks slowly warm, the oxygen evaporates
d. Touching the fill valve can result in burns

28. Which of the following disorders involves sudden or gradual onset of loss of language skills and is characterized by nocturnal multifocal spikes and spike-wave discharges?

a. Temporal lobe epilepsy
b. Lennox-Gastaut syndrome
c. Landau-Kleffner syndrome
d. Dementia with Lewy bodies

29. What is the minimum number of hours that an overnight nocturnal polysomnogram (PSG) should last in order to obtain adequate data?

a. Three
b. Four
c. Five
d. Six

30. Which of the following is FALSE with regard to the multiple sleep latency test (MSLT)?

a. Smoking is not allowed within 30 minutes of starting a nap
b. Physiological calibrations are done five minutes prior to the onset of the nap period
c. A patient should discontinue the use of stimulants two weeks prior to the MSLT
d. The MSLT includes seven nap periods

31. Which of the following is true of supraventricular tachycardia?

a. It originates in the ventricles
b. There may be periods of normal heart rate and rhythm between episodes
c. The QRS complex appears abnormal
d. The P wave is absent

32. Which of the following is NOT true of EEG during stage 2 non-REM sleep?

a. There are periods between K complexes or sleep spindles of less than three minutes that are unrelated to arousal
b. Delta activity is less than 20% of the epoch
c. Abrupt K-complex clusters and delta waves may indicate arousal
d. Activity is high voltage

33. Tidal volume is defined as the

a. amount of air remaining in the lungs after a forced exhalation
b. maximal amount of air exhaled after maximal inhalation
c. amount of air exchange with each breath
d. amount of air in the lungs after a maximal inhalation

34. Which of the following is FALSE with regard to oronasal masks?

a. There is a greater chance of leakage than with nasal masks
b. They cover both the nose and the mouth
c. Nasal pillows must fit snugly into each nostril
d. The masks are often less comfortable for the patient than nasal masks

35. One criterion for scoring pediatric respiratory effort-related arousals (RERAs) is that nasal pressure is reduced by what percentage, compared to baseline?

a. 10%
b. 15%
c. 30%
d. 50%

36. What is the normal range of oxygen saturation?

a. 85-90%
b. 91-94%
c. 95-98%
d. 99-100%

37. Which of the following is true of Cheyne-Stokes respirations?

a. Cheyne-Stokes breathing can occur with damage to the central nervous system (e.g., brain tumor, stroke, traumatic brain injury), hyperventilation, and heart failure
b. Pulse oximetry during the respirations shows a wave-like waveform as saturation begins to rise during the apneic period and then falls after the periods of rapid respirations
c. One criterion for scoring the respirations is the presence of consecutive cycles of a crescendo-to-decrescendo breathing pattern that lasts for a minimum of two consecutive minutes
d. One criterion for scoring the respirations is the presence of consecutive cycles of a crescendo-to-decrescendo breathing pattern that includes three central apneas or central hypopneas per hour of sleep

38. What is the total daily sleep requirement (including both nighttime sleep and daytime naps) for a two-year-old infant?

a. 9.5 hours
b. 10.25 hours
c. 11 hours
d. 13 hours

39. According to proper discharge procedures, after a sleep study has been completed, the technologist should soak and air-dry which of the following pieces of equipment?

a. Snap electrodes
b. Continuous positive airway pressure mask
c. Snore microphone
d. Body position sensors

40. Which of the following is NOT a therapeutic intervention for narcolepsy?

a. Selective serotonin reuptake inhibitors (SSRIs)
b. Methylphenidate
c. Tricyclic antidepressants (TCAs)
d. Controlling obesity by diet and exercise

41. Which of the following actions by the sleep technician violates the principles of proper body mechanics?

a. Avoiding pushing with the arms
b. Avoiding twisting to lift
c. Using a step stool to reach items
d. Bending at the waist to reach items

42. Which of the following neurotransmitters is increased during the awake state; decreased during stages 1, 2, and 3 non-REM sleep; and absent during REM sleep?

a. Serotonin
b. Norepinephrine
c. Glycine
d. Acetylcholine

43. Which of the following is part of the Centers for Disease Control's isolation guidelines?

a. Maintaining a distance of at least 15 feet from a coughing person when possible
b. Using sterile single-use needles and syringes multiple times
c. Washing hands after contact with respiratory secretions
d. Using hand sanitizer after each patient contact

44. In communicating with deaf patients, the interviewer should

a. announce his or her presence by speaking, to see if the patient can lip-read
b. face the interpreter
c. eat when speaking to the patients
d. do none of the above

45. Sleep efficiency is defined as

a. the amount of time needed to go from an awake state to a sleep state
b. the ratio of the percentage of time spent sleeping to the time spent in bed
c. total sleep in minutes for all stages of sleep
d. total minutes spent awake after first falling asleep and until the final awakening time

46. A normal sinus rhythm is characterized by a P wave and QRS complex present with each beat, having a QRS interval of

a. 0.04-0.11 seconds
b. 0.15-0.25 seconds
c. 0.2-0.9 seconds
d. 2-3 seconds

47. Sinus bradycardia is characterized by all of the following EXCEPT

a. a regular pulse of less than 50–60 beats/min with P waves in front of QRS complexes
b. a P-R interval of 0.06–0.12 seconds
c. a QRS interval of 0.04–0.11 seconds
d. a P:QRS ratio of 1:1

48. The Berlin questionnaire (1996) asks about which of the following?

a. Daytime tiredness or fatigue: presence, frequency, and occurrences while driving (falling asleep)
b. Hypertension
c. Snoring: presence, characteristics, frequency, impact on bed partner and others, and apneic episodes
d. All of the above

49. Central sleep apnea is characterized by which of the following?

a. Increased oxygen saturation
b. Absence of chest wall and abdominal movements during apneic periods
c. Snoring that is usually very loud
d. All of the above

50. Dopamine agonists, opioids, anticonvulsants, and benzodiazepines are therapeutic interventions for

a. restless legs syndrome
b. obstructive sleep apnea
c. insomnia
d. circadian rhythm sleep disorder

Answer Key and Explanations

1. A: The correct answer is that total sleep time (TST) decreases to pre-pregnancy levels. Slow-wave sleep (SWS) is normal during the second trimester of pregnancy. REM sleep decreases during the third, not the second, trimester of pregnancy. Shortness of breath increases, not decreases, during the second trimester of pregnancy.

2. A: The correct answer is cardiac output. Cardiac output, which is usually calculated in liters per minute, is the amount of blood that is pumped through the ventricles. Normal cardiac output is about 5 L/min for an adult at rest. Pulmonary vascular resistance (PVR) is the resistance in the pulmonary arteries and arterioles against which the right ventricle has to pump during contraction. PVR is the mean pressure in the pulmonary vascular bed divided by the blood flow. Stroke volume (SV) is the amount of blood pumped through the left ventricle with each contraction, minus any blood that remains inside the ventricle at the end of systole. Normal SV values are 60–70 mL. Cardiac index (CI) is the cardiac output divided by the body surface area (BSA).

3. B: The correct answer is excessive fragmentary myoclonus (EFM). Scoring requires that the activity continue for at least 20 minutes of non-REM sleep, with at least five EMG potentials per minute. EFM appears to be benign. The duration of an activity burst is usually 150 ms or less, but it may be greater than 150 ms if twitching is obvious. By contrast, bruxism is the grinding of the teeth. In REM sleep behavior disorder *(RBD)*, some transient muscle activity (usually involving the muscles of the hands, feet, or mouth) often occurs during REM sleep. In addition, some large muscle activity may occur, but does not involve muscle activity across joints. Rhythmic movement disorder (RMD) is common in infants beginning at approximately six months of age and continuing until two to three years of age; it is rare after age five unless a patient has a central nervous system injury. It often includes rocking, head rolling, or head banging. Some children may also have leg banging and body rolling. Most often, RMD occurs either during stage W, when the patient is very drowsy, or during stage 1 non-REM sleep. The rhythmic movements may be accompanied by humming.

4. B: The purpose of the American Sleep Apnea Association's A.W.A.K.E. program is to educate people about sleep apnea, in order to enable them to manage their health and to provide guidance and ongoing support. It is a program comprised of self-help groups. Groups are advised to be sponsored by a sleep professional (although this is not a requirement). A coordinator leads the meetings, and guest speakers are often invited to speak on topics of interest to the group. ASAA provides suggested meeting topics, and groups meet from monthly to quarterly. In addition, ASAA provides educational material (e.g., newsletters, reports, or videos). A.W.A.K.E. does <u>not</u> provide specialized training to future sleep technologists, diagnose sleep apnea, or fit sleep apnea patients with continuous positive airway pressure masks.

5. C: The cEMG is the chin electromyogram. By recording the muscle tone of the chin muscles, it helps the observer to identify REM sleep (during which there is a reduced muscle tone). The cEMG provides information about snoring, which causes artifacts on cEMG. In addition, it provides information on teeth grinding, which causes muscular movement. It is the EEG (not the cEMG) that provides information on the electrical activity within the brain. Through the use of scalp electrodes, the EEG measures electrical brain activity in order to rule out seizure disorders and to determine sleep-wake state characteristics.

6. C: The correct answer is that if one is not asleep within 20 minutes of going to bed, he or she should get up to do something relaxing until feeling sleepy. According to the principles of good sleep hygiene, the bed should only be used for sleeping and sex. Good sleep hygiene involves avoiding activities that interfere with sleep, such as smoking, drinking alcohol or caffeinated beverages, watching TV in bed right before trying to go to sleep, and taking naps during the day.

7. A: The correct answer is that atrial fibrillation is characterized by a very irregular pulse with an atrial rate of 300-600 beats/minute and a ventricular rate of 120-200 beats/minute. The QRS complex is normal in shape and duration. Fibrillatory (F) waves are present rather than P waves. In addition, the P:QRS ratio is highly variable.

8. A: The correct answer is increased stage 1 non-REM sleep. In a patient with generalized anxiety disorder, polysomnography shows increased stage 1 non-REM sleep, decreased REM density, and a delay in sleep onset.

9. A: The hypothalamus has a role in almost all body processes, including autonomic functions, homeostasis, endocrine processes, emotions, and the regulation of sleep. By contrast, mamillary bodies are active in the memory of smells. The hippocampus is a brain region that is responsible for organizing and processing memories and spatial relationships, and for regulating emotions. The posterior pituitary gland stores and secretes oxytocin and antidiuretic hormone.

10. D: The reservoir should be rinsed thoroughly with water or a vinegar solution and then air-dried. Only distilled water (not tap water) should be used for humidification. The use of tap water may erode the heating element. Proper humidifier care includes emptying the water reservoir each day (not once per week) and washing the reservoir in warm, soapy water (not with bleach).

11. B: The correct answer is that morning/evening questionnaires ask the patient to indicate the five consecutive hours during the day that the patient would prefer to work. A morning/evening questionnaire asks the patient to indicate how he or she feels in the morning after going to sleep at 11 PM. In addition, it asks the patient to assess his or her appetite one-half hour after awakening.

12. B: The hematocrit measures the percentage of packed red blood cells (not white blood cells) in 100 mL of blood. A decrease in the hematocrit can be indicative of anemia, and an increase can be indicative of dehydration. Hematocrit measurements may be used to monitor the effects of rehydration. For men, normal hematocrit values are 42%-52%. For women, normal hematocrit values are 37%-48%.

13. D: The correct answer is 90%. One criterion for scoring pediatric obstructive sleep apnea is that there is a 90% or greater decrease in amplitude for 90% or more of events, compared to baseline.

14. A: The correct answer is generalized tonic-clonic seizures. Generalized tonic-clonic seizures may affect part of or the entire brain. Interictal epileptiform activity (IEA) refers to epileptic-like changes in the EEG that commonly occur between seizures and during sleep. Primary generalized myoclonic epilepsy is characterized by brief jerking motions. Amyotrophic lateral sclerosis (ALS) is a degenerative disease of the motor neurons from the anterior horns of the spinal cord and the motor nuclei in the lower brainstem. ALS is characterized by increasing muscle weakness, spasticity, twitching, fatigue, and lack of coordination. The symptoms of West syndrome include brain damage, resulting in infantile spasms, intellectual disability, and interictal EEG hypsarrhythmia.

15. D: A type 2 sleep study is a modified home sleep study (not one occurring at a sleep center), using portable devices. A type 2 sleep study must include the following seven information channels: EEG, ECG, EOG, EMG, pulse oximetry, respiratory effort, and airflow sensors.

16. D: The correct answer is 9-35. The Fatigue Severity Scale contains nine statements related to fatigue. The patient is required to score each statement on a scale of 1 to 7 (in which 1 is *strongly disagree* and 7 is *strongly agree*). Examples of the statements include: "I become fatigued easily," "I cannot adequately carry out all of my duties and responsibilities because of fatigue," and "My work, social, and family life suffer because of my fatigue." The scores for each statement are added together, with a score between 9 and 35 considered to be in the normal range. Scores above 35 suggest a high degree of fatigue.

17. C: The correct answer is that missed respirations are associated with arousal, awakening, or desaturation of 3% or more. Answers A, B, and D are included in scoring pediatric obstructive sleep apnea. The scoring for central sleep apnea includes a duration of 20 or more seconds or a duration of two or more missed respirations (or equivalent), associated with arousal, awakening, or desaturation of 3% or more.

18. D: The correct answer is diabetic ketoacidosis (DKA). DKA is a complication of diabetes mellitus. Since insulin is not produced adequately, glucose is unavailable for metabolism. As a result, lipolysis produces free fatty acids as an alternate fuel source. Glycerol in fat cells and the liver is converted to ketone bodies, which are used for cellular metabolism less efficiently than glucose. The ketone bodies lower the pH of serum, which leads to ketoacidosis. By contrast, myocardial infarction (MI) occurs when there is an imbalance between the supply and demand of oxygen for the heart. An acute asthma attack is brought upon by some stimulus (e.g., an antigen that triggers an allergic response). This results in an inflammatory cascade that causes a swollen airway, contraction of smooth muscles, increased mucous production, and airway hyperinflation. Strokes result from an interruption in blood flow to a region of the brain.

19. D: The materials should be written at a level that is not higher than a 6th to 8th grade level. Regardless of educational level achieved, the average American reads effectively at the 6th to 8th grade level. Readability index calculators, which provide an approximation of grade level and difficulty for reading materials, are available online.

20. C: The correct answer is central sleep apnea. Patients with pseudohypertrophic Duchenne muscular dystrophy typically have obstructive sleep apnea, not central sleep apnea. Typical problems include hypercapnia and oxygen desaturation during REM sleep, progressing to non-REM sleep as the condition worsens. More typical problems include a decrease in vital capacity to less than 2 L and increasing sleep disruption.

21. B: The correct answer is beta waves. Delta waves are slow waves (1–4 Hz), with an amplitude of more than 75 μV, and are present in stage 3 non-REM (slow-wave) sleep in adults. Delta waves occur in the waking state of newborns and young children and may occur in adults who are intoxicated or have schizophrenia or dementia. Vertex waves are commonly found negative deflections, with amplitude typically ranging from 50–150 μV. Vertex waves are most noticeable from the vertex and frontal leads. They may have sharp contours and occur in repetitive episodes (particularly in children). By contrast, theta waves have a frequency of 4–6 Hz and oscillations of varying amplitude, and are most easily seen with central and temporal leads. Theta waves frequently occur during daydreaming and self-hypnotic states, occur in stage 1 non-REM sleep, and may occur during arousals.

22. C: The correct answer is high impedance. A skin rash can change the skin's electrical signal. When this occurs, the technician should reposition the electrode, avoiding the irritated skin. By contrast, vibration may cause high-frequency artifacts. Swallowing can result in slow waves on EEG, and the blink produces slow waves on EOG. Eye muscle abnormality can cause a spike on EEG.

23. A: Pulse oximetry measures arterial oxygen saturation (SpO_2). By contrast, anterior tibialis electromyograms (atEMGs) monitor electrical activity in the leg muscles. When the leg muscles are relaxed, electrical activity is not present. With movement, electrical activity increases. The EOG records both vertical and horizontal eye movements and helps the observer to identify periods of REM sleep. Microphones or piezo sensors are used to indicate the degree and duration of snoring.

24. D: Statements A-C are all true. Periodic limb movements of sleep are scored as either events or series. It is a series (not an event) that requires four or more consecutive leg movements with the interval between movements ranging from 5-90 seconds. Leg movements that involve both legs are counted as one movement if they occur within 5 seconds of one another.

25. D: As air becomes cooler, its ability to hold water decreases. As a result, condensation begins to form in the tubing. This causes audible gurgling and decreased pressure, which are important to avoid in order for effective therapy to occur. One solution is to increase (not decrease) the room temperature by 5 to 6 degrees at night. Other potential solutions include using heated tubing and reducing the level of humidification. Another potential solution is to insulate the tubing to reduce the effects of ambient temperature.

26. C: The impedance levels for each individual electrode should be less than or equal to 5 kΩ. Electrodes should be tested individually (not in groups of three) with an internal impedance meter or an external handheld meter. When there is a difference in impedance between electrodes, it increases artifacts. The sleep technologist should verify the electrode impedances after calibrating the machine.

27. B: Liquid oxygen is maintained at 21 psi, not 18 psi. It is true that it is stored at temperatures of -183°C in special cryogenic containers that oxygen evaporates as the tanks slowly warm, and that touching the fill valve can result in burns.

28. C: Landau-Kleffner syndrome involves sudden or gradual onset of loss of language skills and is characterized by nocturnal multifocal spikes and spike-wave discharges. Temporal lobe epilepsy is characterized by an increase in interictal epileptiform activity (IEA) in non-REM sleep with high-frequency spikes and contralateral focal discharges. It is also characterized by a reduction in REM sleep. Lennox-Gastaut syndrome is an intractable seizure disorder characterized by many kinds of seizures, which occur throughout waking and sleeping, and by intellectual disability. Dementia with Lewy bodies is characterized by cognitive and physical decline, with symptoms that fluctuate often. A primary feature on polysomnography is REM behavior disorder.

29. D: The correct answer is six hours or more. It is necessary to note the exact start and stop time for the polysomnogram (PSG). Insurance may not pay for an incomplete PSG, so all interruptions should be noted (e.g., an emergency that necessitates ending the study early).

30. D: The multiple sleep latency test (MSLT) includes five nap periods, not seven. The first nap period is within three hours of a nocturnal polysomnogram, and then spaced at two hours after the beginning of the preceding nap. It is true that the patient must not smoke within 30 minutes of starting a nap and that physiological calibrations are performed five minutes prior to the onset of the nap period. Also, a patient should stop using stimulants two weeks prior to the MSLT, so that the stimulants do not interfere with the results of the test.

31. B: The correct answer is that supraventricular tachycardia may be episodic, with periods of normal heart rate and rhythm between episodes. It originates in the atria, not the ventricles. The QRS complex appears normal. The P wave is present, but it may not be clearly defined since it may be obscured by the preceding T wave.

32. D: Stage 2 non-REM sleep is characterized on EEG by low-voltage (not high-voltage) activity with mixed frequency. Stage 2 is characterized by intervening periods between K complexes or sleep spindles of less than three minutes that are unrelated to arousal. Delta activity is less than 20% of the epoch. Also, normal K-complex activity is 1–3 per minute in young adults. Arousal may be indicated by abrupt K-complex clusters and delta waves.

33. C: *Tidal volume* is the amount of air exchange with each breath. *Residual volume* is the amount of air remaining in the lungs after a forced exhalation. *Vital capacity* is the maximal amount of air exhaled after maximal inhalation. *Total lung capacity* is the amount of air in the lungs after a maximal inhalation.

34. C: For patients who use nasal masks (as opposed to oronasal masks), nasal pillows must fit snugly into each nostril. With oronasal masks, there is a greater chance of air leakage than with nasal masks. Oronasal masks cover both the nose and the mouth, so they are often more effective than nasal masks. However, oronasal masks are often less comfortable for the patient than nasal masks.

35. C: The correct answer is that one criterion for scoring pediatric respiratory effort-related arousals is that there is a 30% or more reduction in nasal pressure, compared to baseline. Additional scoring criteria for nasal pressure are a flattening of nasal pressure waveforms; evidence of snoring, snoring respirations, increased carbon dioxide partial pressure (pCO2), or observable increased respiratory effort; and a duration of two or more respirations (or an equivalent duration of two respirations based upon baseline recordings).

36. C: The correct answer is 95-98% oxygen saturation. This is equal to a normal PaO_2 of 80–100 mm Hg. Levels that are lower than 40 mm Hg are dangerous.

37. A: The correct answer is that Cheyne-Strokes breathing can occur with damage to the central nervous system, hyperventilation, and heart failure. Pulse oximetry during the respirations shows a wave-like waveform as saturation begins to fall during the apneic period and then rises during periods of rapid respirations. One criterion for scoring the respirations is consecutive cycles of a crescendo-to-decrescendo breathing pattern that lasts for a minimum of ten (not two) consecutive minutes. One criterion for scoring the respirations is consecutive cycles of a crescendo-to-decrescendo breathing pattern that include five (not three) central apneas or central hypopneas per hour of sleep.

38. D: The correct answer is 13 hours. A five-year-old child requires 11 hours, and an eight-year-old child requires 10.25 hours. An eleven-year-old child requires a daily 9.5 hours of sleep.

39. B: The correct answer is the continuous positive airway pressure mask. This mask must be soaked (not just wiped clean) and air-dried. The other equipment listed (snap electrodes, snore microphone, and body position sensors) must be wiped clean (not soaked) and air-dried.

40. D: Controlling obesity by diet and exercise is a therapeutic intervention for obstructive sleep apnea (OSA), but not for narcolepsy. OSA symptoms tend to lessen with weight loss. By contrast, selective serotonin reuptake inhibitors (SSRIs) and tricyclic antidepressants (TCAs) are therapeutic interventions for narcolepsy. Amphetamine-like drugs such as methylphenidate decrease sleepiness during the daytime and reduce daytime sleeping.

41. D: The correct answer is bending at the waist to reach items. Such bending should be avoided; rather, the technician should stoop down with the knees bent. It is very important for sleep technicians to use proper body mechanics, in order to prevent back injury when helping patients to change positions during the night. It is important to avoid pushing or pulling with the arms. Instead, the technician should use the entire body to relieve strain on the arms and back. Furthermore, the technician should use a step stool to reach items that are out of reach (as opposed to stretching overhead). Rather than twisting to lift, the technician should stand near the person or item to be lifted, bend his or her knees and hips, and use the muscles in his or her legs to support weight rather than using his or her back or arms to support the weight.

42. B: The correct answer is norepinephrine. In order to maintain the awake state, levels of norepinephrine increase. Levels of norepinephrine decrease during stages 1, 2, and 3 non-REM sleep. During REM sleep, norepinephrine is absent. Serotonin levels rise during the awake state but decrease during non-REM and REM sleep. This helps to regulate the onset of sleep, with the lowest levels present during REM sleep. During REM sleep, glycine levels rise to inhibit the motor nervous system at the spinal cord to cause atonia. Acetylcholine levels rise during the wake state and during REM sleep, and decrease during stages 1, 2, and 3 non-REM sleep.

43. C: The isolation guidelines include washing hands after contact with respiratory secretions. The isolation guidelines include washing hands, not using hand sanitizer, after each patient contact. Additional guidelines include maintaining a distance of three feet or more from a coughing person when possible (to avoid inhaling respiratory droplets) and using sterile single-use needles and syringes one time only.

44. D: The correct answer is *none of the above*. Deaf individuals rely on visual and sensory cues to know when someone is in the room, so the interviewer should announce his or her presence in the room by waving, clapping, or tapping the foot. The interviewer should always face the patient, not the interpreter. Also, it is important etiquette to refrain from eating when speaking to the patients.

45. B: *Sleep efficiency* (SE) is defined as the ratio of the percentage of time spent sleeping to the time spent in bed. *Sleep onset latency* (SOL) determines the amount of time needed to go from an awake state to a sleep state. *Total sleep time* (TST) is defined as the total sleep in minutes for all stages of sleep. *Wake-after sleep onset* (WASO) is defined as the total minutes spent awake after first falling asleep and until the final awakening time.

46. A: The correct answer is 0.04-0.11 seconds. In addition, a normal sinus rhythm is characterized by each beat having a P:QRS ratio of 1:1 and a P-R interval of 0.12–0.20 seconds.

47. B: Sinus bradycardia is characterized by a P-R interval of 0.12-0.20 seconds (not 0.06-0.12 seconds). It is true that sinus bradycardia is characterized by a regular pulse of less than 50–60 beats/min with P waves in front of QRS complexes, which are usually normal in shape and duration; a QRS interval of 0.04–0.11 seconds; and a P:QRS ratio of 1:1.

48. D: The correct answer is *all of the above*. The Berlin questionnaire (1996) is most often used for screening people who are at risk for obstructive sleep apnea (OSA). Occasionally, it is used to assess a patient's progress after the onset of treatment with positive airway pressure. The questionnaire contains a total of fourteen questions in three categories. The questions in category 1 assess snoring (presence, characteristics, frequency, impact on bed partner and others, and apneic episodes). The questions in category 2 assess daytime tiredness or fatigue: presence, frequency, and occurrences while driving (falling asleep). The questions in category 3 assess whether hypertension is present or body mass index (BMI) is 30 kg/m^2 or more. A patient is classified as *high risk* or *low risk* based upon positive findings in the three different categories. A patient who is classified as high risk is one for whom positive scores are found in two or three categories. A patient who is considered low risk is one for whom positive scores are found in no more than one category.

49. B: In central sleep apnea, apneic episodes occur without obstruction of the upper airway. Central sleep apnea typically results from neurological or cardiac disorders that cause impairment of ventilation. In central sleep apnea, reduced oxygen saturation is present. There is an absence of chest wall and abdominal movements during the apneic periods. Snoring is usually mild (as opposed to obstructive sleep apnea, which is characterized by loud snoring).

50. A: The correct answer is restless legs syndrome (RLS). Dopamine agonists, opioids, and anticonvulsants may reduce symptoms of RLS. The benzodiazepine clonazepam depresses central nervous system activity; it allows the patient to sleep more but does not fully eradicate RLS.

How to Overcome Test Anxiety

Just the thought of taking a test is enough to make most people a little nervous. A test is an important event that can have a long-term impact on your future, so it's important to take it seriously and it's natural to feel anxious about performing well. But just because anxiety is normal, that doesn't mean that it's helpful in test taking, or that you should simply accept it as part of your life. Anxiety can have a variety of effects. These effects can be mild, like making you feel slightly nervous, or severe, like blocking your ability to focus or remember even a simple detail.

If you experience test anxiety—whether severe or mild—it's important to know how to beat it. To discover this, first you need to understand what causes test anxiety.

Causes of Test Anxiety

While we often think of anxiety as an uncontrollable emotional state, it can actually be caused by simple, practical things. One of the most common causes of test anxiety is that a person does not feel adequately prepared for their test. This feeling can be the result of many different issues such as poor study habits or lack of organization, but the most common culprit is time management. Starting to study too late, failing to organize your study time to cover all of the material, or being distracted while you study will mean that you're not well prepared for the test. This may lead to cramming the night before, which will cause you to be physically and mentally exhausted for the test. Poor time management also contributes to feelings of stress, fear, and hopelessness as you realize you are not well prepared but don't know what to do about it.

Other times, test anxiety is not related to your preparation for the test but comes from unresolved fear. This may be a past failure on a test, or poor performance on tests in general. It may come from comparing yourself to others who seem to be performing better or from the stress of living up to expectations. Anxiety may be driven by fears of the future—how failure on this test would affect your educational and career goals. These fears are often completely irrational, but they can still negatively impact your test performance.

Elements of Test Anxiety

As mentioned earlier, test anxiety is considered to be an emotional state, but it has physical and mental components as well. Sometimes you may not even realize that you are suffering from test anxiety until you notice the physical symptoms. These can include trembling hands, rapid heartbeat, sweating, nausea, and tense muscles. Extreme anxiety may lead to fainting or vomiting. Obviously, any of these symptoms can have a negative impact on testing. It is important to recognize them as soon as they begin to occur so that you can address the problem before it damages your performance.

The mental components of test anxiety include trouble focusing and inability to remember learned information. During a test, your mind is on high alert, which can help you recall information and stay focused for an extended period of time. However, anxiety interferes with your mind's natural processes, causing you to blank out, even on the questions you know well. The strain of testing during anxiety makes it difficult to stay focused, especially on a test that may take several hours. Extreme anxiety can take a huge mental toll, making it difficult not only to recall test information but even to understand the test questions or pull your thoughts together.

Effects of Test Anxiety

Test anxiety is like a disease—if left untreated, it will get progressively worse. Anxiety leads to poor performance, and this reinforces the feelings of fear and failure, which in turn lead to poor performances on subsequent tests. It can grow from a mild nervousness to a crippling condition. If allowed to progress, test anxiety can have a big impact on your schooling, and consequently on your future.

Test anxiety can spread to other parts of your life. Anxiety on tests can become anxiety in any stressful situation, and blanking on a test can turn into panicking in a job situation. But fortunately, you don't have to let anxiety rule your testing and determine your grades. There are a number of relatively simple steps you can take to move past anxiety and function normally on a test and in the rest of life.

Physical Steps for Beating Test Anxiety

While test anxiety is a serious problem, the good news is that it can be overcome. It doesn't have to control your ability to think and remember information. While it may take time, you can begin taking steps today to beat anxiety.

Just as your first hint that you may be struggling with anxiety comes from the physical symptoms, the first step to treating it is also physical. Rest is crucial for having a clear, strong mind. If you are tired, it is much easier to give in to anxiety. But if you establish good sleep habits, your body and mind will be ready to perform optimally, without the strain of exhaustion. Additionally, sleeping well helps you to retain information better, so you're more likely to recall the answers when you see the test questions.

Getting good sleep means more than going to bed on time. It's important to allow your brain time to relax. Take study breaks from time to time so it doesn't get overworked, and don't study right before bed. Take time to rest your mind before trying to rest your body, or you may find it difficult to fall asleep.

Along with sleep, other aspects of physical health are important in preparing for a test. Good nutrition is vital for good brain function. Sugary foods and drinks may give a burst of energy but this burst is followed by a crash, both physically and emotionally. Instead, fuel your body with protein and vitamin-rich foods.

Also, drink plenty of water. Dehydration can lead to headaches and exhaustion, especially if your brain is already under stress from the rigors of the test. Particularly if your test is a long one, drink water during the breaks. And if possible, take an energy-boosting snack to eat between sections.

Along with sleep and diet, a third important part of physical health is exercise. Maintaining a steady workout schedule is helpful, but even taking 5-minute study breaks to walk can help get your blood pumping faster and clear your head. Exercise also releases endorphins, which contribute to a positive feeling and can help combat test anxiety.

When you nurture your physical health, you are also contributing to your mental health. If your body is healthy, your mind is much more likely to be healthy as well. So take time to rest, nourish your body with healthy food and water, and get moving as much as possible. Taking these physical steps will make you stronger and more able to take the mental steps necessary to overcome test anxiety.

Mental Steps for Beating Test Anxiety

Working on the mental side of test anxiety can be more challenging, but as with the physical side, there are clear steps you can take to overcome it. As mentioned earlier, test anxiety often stems from lack of preparation, so the obvious solution is to prepare for the test. Effective studying may be the most important weapon you have for beating test anxiety, but you can and should employ several other mental tools to combat fear.

First, boost your confidence by reminding yourself of past success—tests or projects that you aced. If you're putting as much effort into preparing for this test as you did for those, there's no reason you should expect to fail here. Work hard to prepare; then trust your preparation.

Second, surround yourself with encouraging people. It can be helpful to find a study group, but be sure that the people you're around will encourage a positive attitude. If you spend time with others who are anxious or cynical, this will only contribute to your own anxiety. Look for others who are motivated to study hard from a desire to succeed, not from a fear of failure.

Third, reward yourself. A test is physically and mentally tiring, even without anxiety, and it can be helpful to have something to look forward to. Plan an activity following the test, regardless of the outcome, such as going to a movie or getting ice cream.

When you are taking the test, if you find yourself beginning to feel anxious, remind yourself that you know the material. Visualize successfully completing the test. Then take a few deep, relaxing breaths and return to it. Work through the questions carefully but with confidence, knowing that you are capable of succeeding.

Developing a healthy mental approach to test taking will also aid in other areas of life. Test anxiety affects more than just the actual test—it can be damaging to your mental health and even contribute to depression. It's important to beat test anxiety before it becomes a problem for more than testing.

Study Strategy

Being prepared for the test is necessary to combat anxiety, but what does being prepared look like? You may study for hours on end and still not feel prepared. What you need is a strategy for test prep. The next few pages outline our recommended steps to help you plan out and conquer the challenge of preparation.

Step 1: Scope Out the Test

Learn everything you can about the format (multiple choice, essay, etc.) and what will be on the test. Gather any study materials, course outlines, or sample exams that may be available. Not only will this help you to prepare, but knowing what to expect can help to alleviate test anxiety.

Step 2: Map Out the Material

Look through the textbook or study guide and make note of how many chapters or sections it has. Then divide these over the time you have. For example, if a book has 15 chapters and you have five days to study, you need to cover three chapters each day. Even better, if you have the time, leave an extra day at the end for overall review after you have gone through the material in depth.

If time is limited, you may need to prioritize the material. Look through it and make note of which sections you think you already have a good grasp on, and which need review. While you are studying, skim quickly through the familiar sections and take more time on the challenging parts.

Write out your plan so you don't get lost as you go. Having a written plan also helps you feel more in control of the study, so anxiety is less likely to arise from feeling overwhelmed at the amount to cover.

Step 3: Gather Your Tools

Decide what study method works best for you. Do you prefer to highlight in the book as you study and then go back over the highlighted portions? Or do you type out notes of the important information? Or is it helpful to make flashcards that you can carry with you? Assemble the pens, index cards, highlighters, post-it notes, and any other materials you may need so you won't be distracted by getting up to find things while you study.

If you're having a hard time retaining the information or organizing your notes, experiment with different methods. For example, try color-coding by subject with colored pens, highlighters, or post-it notes. If you learn better by hearing, try recording yourself reading your notes so you can listen while in the car, working out, or simply sitting at your desk. Ask a friend to quiz you from your flashcards, or try teaching someone the material to solidify it in your mind.

Step 4: Create Your Environment

It's important to avoid distractions while you study. This includes both the obvious distractions like visitors and the subtle distractions like an uncomfortable chair (or a too-comfortable couch that makes you want to fall asleep). Set up the best study environment possible: good lighting and a comfortable work area. If background music helps you focus, you may want to turn it on, but otherwise keep the room quiet. If you are using a computer to take notes, be sure you don't have any other windows open, especially applications like social media, games, or anything else that could distract you. Silence your phone and turn off notifications. Be sure to keep water close by so you stay hydrated while you study (but avoid unhealthy drinks and snacks).

Also, take into account the best time of day to study. Are you freshest first thing in the morning? Try to set aside some time then to work through the material. Is your mind clearer in the afternoon or evening? Schedule your study session then. Another method is to study at the same time of day that you will take the test, so that your brain gets used to working on the material at that time and will be ready to focus at test time.

Step 5: Study!

Once you have done all the study preparation, it's time to settle into the actual studying. Sit down, take a few moments to settle your mind so you can focus, and begin to follow your study plan. Don't give in to distractions or let yourself procrastinate. This is your time to prepare so you'll be ready to fearlessly approach the test. Make the most of the time and stay focused.

Of course, you don't want to burn out. If you study too long you may find that you're not retaining the information very well. Take regular study breaks. For example, taking five minutes out of every hour to walk briskly, breathing deeply and swinging your arms, can help your mind stay fresh.

As you get to the end of each chapter or section, it's a good idea to do a quick review. Remind yourself of what you learned and work on any difficult parts. When you feel that you've mastered the material, move on to the next part. At the end of your study session, briefly skim through your notes again.

But while review is helpful, cramming last minute is NOT. If at all possible, work ahead so that you won't need to fit all your study into the last day. Cramming overloads your brain with more information than it can process and retain, and your tired mind may struggle to recall even previously learned information when it is overwhelmed with last-minute study. Also, the urgent nature of cramming and the stress placed on your brain contribute to anxiety. You'll be more likely to go to the test feeling unprepared and having trouble thinking clearly.

So don't cram, and don't stay up late before the test, even just to review your notes at a leisurely pace. Your brain needs rest more than it needs to go over the information again. In fact, plan to finish your studies by noon or early afternoon the day before the test. Give your brain the rest of the day to relax or focus on other things, and get a good night's sleep. Then you will be fresh for the test and better able to recall what you've studied.

Step 6: Take a Practice Test

Many courses offer sample tests, either online or in the study materials. This is an excellent resource to check whether you have mastered the material, as well as to prepare for the test format and environment.

Check the test format ahead of time: the number of questions, the type (multiple choice, free response, etc.), and the time limit. Then create a plan for working through them. For example, if you have 30 minutes to take a 60-question test, your limit is 30 seconds per question. Spend less time on the questions you know well so that you can take more time on the difficult ones.

If you have time to take several practice tests, take the first one open book, with no time limit. Work through the questions at your own pace and make sure you fully understand them. Gradually work up to taking a test under test conditions: sit at a desk with all study materials put away and set a timer. Pace yourself to make sure you finish the test with time to spare and go back to check your answers if you have time.

After each test, check your answers. On the questions you missed, be sure you understand why you missed them. Did you misread the question (tests can use tricky wording)? Did you forget the information? Or was it something you hadn't learned? Go back and study any shaky areas that the practice tests reveal.

Taking these tests not only helps with your grade, but also aids in combating test anxiety. If you're already used to the test conditions, you're less likely to worry about it, and working through tests until you're scoring well gives you a confidence boost. Go through the practice tests until you feel comfortable, and then you can go into the test knowing that you're ready for it.

Test Tips

On test day, you should be confident, knowing that you've prepared well and are ready to answer the questions. But aside from preparation, there are several test day strategies you can employ to maximize your performance.

First, as stated before, get a good night's sleep the night before the test (and for several nights before that, if possible). Go into the test with a fresh, alert mind rather than staying up late to study.

Try not to change too much about your normal routine on the day of the test. It's important to eat a nutritious breakfast, but if you normally don't eat breakfast at all, consider eating just a protein bar. If you're a coffee drinker, go ahead and have your normal coffee. Just make sure you time it so that the caffeine doesn't wear off right in the middle of your test. Avoid sugary beverages, and drink enough water to stay hydrated but not so much that you need a restroom break 10 minutes into the test. If your test isn't first thing in the morning, consider going for a walk or doing a light workout before the test to get your blood flowing.

Allow yourself enough time to get ready, and leave for the test with plenty of time to spare so you won't have the anxiety of scrambling to arrive in time. Another reason to be early is to select a good seat. It's helpful to sit away from doors and windows, which can be distracting. Find a good seat, get out your supplies, and settle your mind before the test begins.

When the test begins, start by going over the instructions carefully, even if you already know what to expect. Make sure you avoid any careless mistakes by following the directions.

Then begin working through the questions, pacing yourself as you've practiced. If you're not sure on an answer, don't spend too much time on it, and don't let it shake your confidence. Either skip it and come back later, or eliminate as many wrong answers as possible and guess among the remaining ones. Don't dwell on these questions as you continue—put them out of your mind and focus on what lies ahead.

Be sure to read all of the answer choices, even if you're sure the first one is the right answer. Sometimes you'll find a better one if you keep reading. But don't second-guess yourself if you do immediately know the answer. Your gut instinct is usually right. Don't let test anxiety rob you of the information you know.

If you have time at the end of the test (and if the test format allows), go back and review your answers. Be cautious about changing any, since your first instinct tends to be correct, but make sure you didn't misread any of the questions or accidentally mark the wrong answer choice. Look over any you skipped and make an educated guess.

At the end, leave the test feeling confident. You've done your best, so don't waste time worrying about your performance or wishing you could change anything. Instead, celebrate the successful completion of this test. And finally, use this test to learn how to deal with anxiety even better next time.

Review Video: Test Anxiety
Visit mometrix.com/academy and enter code: 100340

Important Qualification

Not all anxiety is created equal. If your test anxiety is causing major issues in your life beyond the classroom or testing center, or if you are experiencing troubling physical symptoms related to your anxiety, it may be a sign of a serious physiological or psychological condition. If this sounds like your situation, we strongly encourage you to seek professional help.

Online Resources

Due to our efforts to try to keep this book to a manageable length, we've created a link that will give you access to all of your online resources:

mometrix.com/resources719/regsleeptech

It's Your Moment, Let's Celebrate It!

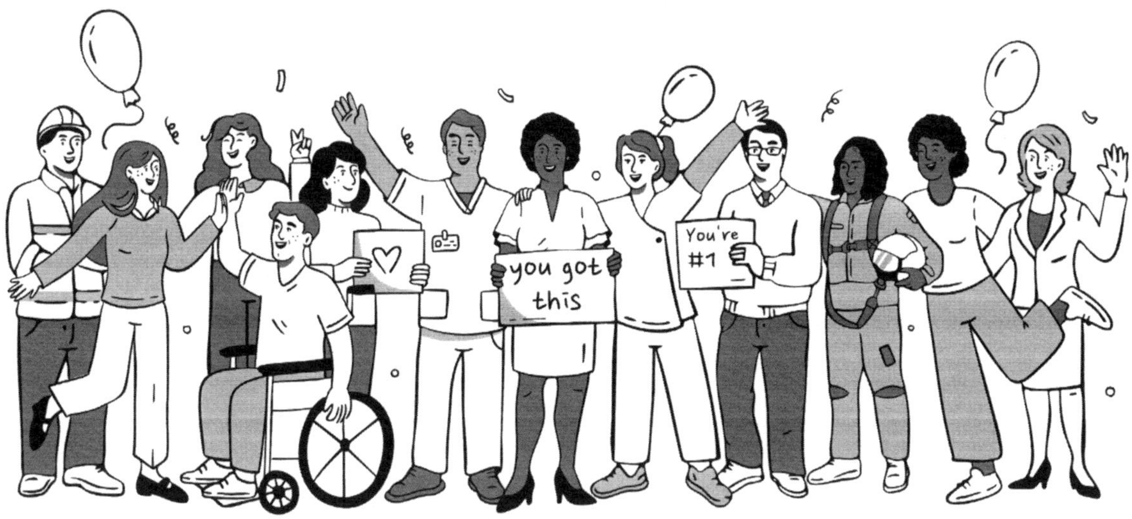

Share your story @mometrixtestpreparation